JOANN C JENNY

The Ultimate Guide to Intermittent Fasting and the Keto Diet

Achieving Optimal Health and Weight with Recipes, a 21-Day Meal Plan, and a 30-Day IF Routine

Contents

II The Power of Intermittent Fasting

III The Ultimate Guide to the Keto Diet:
Achieving Health and Weight Loss

I

Reaching Your Optimal Weight: The Path to a Healthier You

"Embark on your weight loss journey with unwavering determination and watch as your efforts sculpt not just your body, but also the incredible strength of your spirit. Take the plunge into Intermittent Fasting and Keto – your path to the best health and weight begins with a single step."

Introduction

I n a picturesque village tucked away between rolling hills, there lived a man named Marcus. He had a dream - to reach the pinnacle of health and weight. He had heard rumors about the potential of Intermittent Fasting and the Keto Diet, and with a fire in his heart, he set out on a journey that would alter his life forever.

Marcus began his mission by searching for the perfect guide to Intermittent Fasting and the Keto Diet. He traveled far and wide, consulting knowledgeable sages and experienced healers, and taking in all the knowledge they had to offer. With this newfound wisdom, he set up camp at the base of Mount Vitality, ready to start his transformation.

The path ahead was not easy, and Marcus was met with obstacles at every turn. The allure of sugary snacks and hearty meals tested his resolve, but he kept his eye on the prize - optimal health and weight. He embraced Intermittent Fasting, fasting during designated hours, and followed the Keto Diet, replacing carbs with healthy fats and greens.

As time passed, Marcus's body adjusted to this new lifestyle.

He noticed his energy levels rising, his mind becoming sharper, and the extra weight melting away. But it wasn't just physical changes; Marcus felt a sense of accomplishment and empowerment. He had discovered a newfound discipline and inner strength he never knew he had.

As the seasons changed, so did Marcus's journey. He started to share his experiences and the knowledge he had gained with his fellow villagers. He held workshops, led discussions, and encouraged others to begin their own paths to optimal health. The village was transformed, as people adopted Intermittent Fasting and the Keto Diet, finding new vitality and leaving behind years of unhealthy habits.

News of Marcus's success spread beyond the village, reaching the ears of a renowned wellness advocate named Elena. She was intrigued by his story and sought him out to learn more. Elena was deeply impressed by Marcus's unwavering commitment and the positive effect he had on his community.

Together, Marcus and Elena created a comprehensive guide – "The Ultimate Guide to Intermittent Fasting, Keto Diet, and Achieving Optimal Health and Weight." Their collaboration combined ancient wisdom with modern science, providing a roadmap for anyone looking to improve their health and well-being.

The guide became a worldwide sensation, motivating countless people to start their own journeys. Marcus and Elena traveled far and wide, spreading the message of hope, discipline, and self-discovery. Their legacy continued to grow, as people everywhere embraced Intermittent Fasting and the Keto Diet, unlocking the doors to optimal health and weight.

And so, the story of Marcus and his pursuit of optimal health and weight became a legend, a tale of determination, resilience, and the transformative power of Intermittent Fasting and the Keto Diet.

Welcome to "Reaching Your Optimal Weight: The Path to a Healthier You" In this part, we will embark on a journey to help you reach your weight loss goals and develop a healthier lifestyle.

Weight loss is not just about losing pounds; it is a process that involves understanding your body, making informed decisions, and forming sustainable habits. The journey may not be easy, but it will be worth it.

We will explore different aspects of weight loss, from the science of metabolism to the psychology of eating. We will discuss the importance of exercise, the effects of sleep and stress, and how to manage emotional eating.

It is essential to remember that this is not a quick fix. Crash diets and extreme workout plans often lead to short-term results and can be damaging to your health. Instead, we will focus on gradual, lasting changes that will benefit your overall well-being.

By the end of this book, you will have a thorough understanding of what it takes to reach your ideal weight and keep it. You will have the knowledge, tools, and motivation to take control of your health and transform your life.

So, let's start this journey together, embracing the possibilities that lie ahead, and working towards becoming the best version of ourselves.

Chapter 1: The Basics of Weight Loss

I f you're starting a weight loss journey, it's important to have a solid foundation. Before you dive into any diet plans or exercise routines, it's essential to understand the fundamentals of successful weight loss.

Comprehending Calories and Energy Balance

At the core of weight loss is the concept of calories and energy balance. In a nutshell, weight loss happens when you burn more calories than you consume. This creates a calorie deficit, causing your body to use its fat stores for energy.

The first step is to figure out your daily caloric needs. Factors such as age, gender, weight, height, and activity level all affect the number of calories your body needs to stay at its current weight. By eating fewer calories than your maintenance level, you start the weight loss process.

Importance of a Balanced Diet

While a calorie deficit is essential, it's just as important to focus on the quality of the calories you eat. A balanced diet that includes a variety of nutrient-dense foods is essential for overall health and sustainable weight loss.

Try to include plenty of fruits, vegetables, whole grains, lean proteins, and healthy fats in your meals. These provide essential vitamins, minerals, and macronutrients that support your body's functions and keep you feeling full.

The Role of Physical Activity

Regular physical activity is an important part of any weight loss journey. Exercise not only burns calories but also helps to preserve lean muscle mass, which is essential for keeping a healthy metabolism.

Find activities that you enjoy, such as brisk walking, cycling, dancing, or swimming. Consistency is key, so aim for at least 150 minutes of moderate-intensity exercise per week.

Building a Support System

Weight loss can be difficult, and having a support system can make a huge difference. Surround yourself with friends, family, or join a community of people with similar goals. They can give you motivation, encouragement, and accountability throughout your journey.

Conclusion

Having a strong foundation is essential for a successful weight loss journey. By understanding the principles of energy balance, eating a balanced diet, staying physically active, and seeking support, you set yourself up for long-term success.

In Chapter 2, we'll look at the details of understanding your body and metabolism, providing insights that will help you reach a healthier you.

Chapter 2: Understanding Your Body and Metabolism

U nderstanding how your body functions and how metabolism affects weight loss is key if you want to lose weight in a healthy and lasting way. We will go more deeply into the complexities of metabolism and how many things affect it in this chapter.

Metabolism: What Is It?

The chemical reactions that take place in your body to preserve life are referred to as metabolism. It entails the transformation of food into energy, which powers several body processes like respiration, digestion, and cell repair. How effectively your body burns calories is determined by your metabolic rate.

Metabolic Affecting Factors

Your metabolic rate can be affected by several things:

1. Age: As we get older, our metabolism slows down, which results in less calorie burning. Regular exercise, however, can lessen the impact of this.

2. Body Composition: Compared to fat tissue, muscle tissue demands more energy to sustain. As a result, people with a higher ratio of muscle to fat typically have higher metabolic rates.

3. Hormones: Hormones are crucial in controlling metabolism. Particularly thyroid hormones have a direct effect on how effectively calories are burnt.

4. Genetics: Your metabolism may be impacted by your genetic makeup. Different people naturally have different rates of metabolism.

5. Caloric Intake: Your metabolism can slow down if you eat too few calories since your body will go into "starvation mode" to conserve energy.

Increasing Metabolism

There are strategies to improve your metabolism even while some aspects, including age and genetics, are beyond your control:

1. Strength Training: By regularly performing strength training activities, you can build more muscle, which raises your resting metabolic rate.

2. High-Intensity Interval Training (HIIT): HIIT exercises consist of quick bursts of vigorous activity followed by quick rest intervals. Even after a workout, this type of activity helps maintain your metabolism high.

3. Consuming Protein-Rich Foods: Protein requires more energy to digest than fats or carbohydrates do. Protein-rich foods might temporarily increase your metabolism if you eat them.

4. Maintaining Hydration: Dehydration might cause your metabolism to slow down. Make sure to hydrate yourself with water throughout the day.

5. Eating Regular Meals: Skipping meals can cause your metabolic rate to drop. Aim for regular, well-balanced meals and steer clear of extended fasts.

A Myth Regarding "Starvation Mode"

Many people are concerned that restricting calories will cause their metabolism to slow down significantly, triggering the dreaded "starvation mode." The body's inherent survival mechanisms do not activate unless you are extremely undernourished, even though severe calorie restriction might temporarily lower your metabolic rate.

Conclusion

The first step in losing weight is understanding your body and metabolism. You may maximize your body's capacity to burn calories effectively by understanding the elements that affect your metabolic rate and implementing measures to raise it.

In Chapter 3, we'll concentrate on developing a personalized plan that suits your particular requirements and desires and setting reasonable weight reduction goals. Recall that progress, not perfection, is the goal of this trip. If you stick with it, you will eventually notice beneficial changes happening.

Chapter 3: Setting Realistic Weight Loss Goals

A ny successful weight loss journey must start with setting attainable and realistic goals. This chapter will cover the value of goal-setting, how to create SMART goals, and how to maintain motivation while you work toward becoming healthier.

The Importance of Setting Goals

Your weight loss attempts have direction and purpose when you have clear, precise goals. They aid in maintaining attention and aid in accurately tracking your advancement. Setting attainable objectives that take into account your present lifestyle, obligations, and abilities is crucial.

The framework for SMART goals

A tried-and-true technique for establishing goals that are Specific, Measurable, Achievable, Relevant, and Time-bound is the SMART goal framework.

1. Specific: Clearly state your desired weight loss. Avoid generalizations like "lose weight" and instead be specific about how much weight you want to reduce and any areas you want to concentrate on.

2. Measurable: Create specific benchmarks to gauge your success. Measurable goals provide concrete evidence of your accomplishments, whether you're measuring weight loss, inches dropped, or improvements in your level of fitness.

3. Achievable: Make sure your objectives are both challenging and doable. Setting unrealistically high goals can result in dissatisfaction and demotivate. When setting your goals, take into account your lifestyle, available resources, and time restrictions.

4. Relevant: Make sure your objectives are consistent with your overall desire for a better lifestyle. Not only a number on the scale, but your general well-being should improve with weight loss.

5. Time-bound: Establish a deadline for completing your goals. A deadline gives you a sense of urgency and keeps you on course.

Long-term vs. Short-term Objectives

It's crucial to set smaller, more immediate goals in addition to long-term ones for weight loss. These serve as stepping

15

stones toward your final goal and provide you with a feeling of achievement along the way.

For instance, your short-term objective might be to lose 2 pounds per week through a combination of diet and exercise, while your long-term objective would be to drop 50 pounds in six months.

Monitoring Your Development

The key to maintaining motivation and making the required plan modifications is to regularly assess your progress. To record your success, keep a journal, use a weight reduction app, or take pictures.

Celebrate all of your accomplishments, no matter how minor, and take lessons from failures. Remember that obstacles will inevitably arise during any transforming process; what matters most is your resolve to keep going.

Seeking Assistance

enlist the aid of your friends, family, or even a coach or support group for weight loss. Having a companion on your path can offer support, responsibility, and comprehension.

Conclusion

A successful and long-lasting journey to a healthy you starts with setting realistic weight loss objectives. You can strengthen your resolve to stick with it and get beyond challenges by using the SMART goal framework, breaking down your dreams into manageable short-term goals, and monitoring your progress.

In Chapter 4, we'll look at the key elements of designing a wholesome diet that will fuel your body and aid in weight loss. Keep in mind that each step you take will get you one step closer to achieving your objective.

Chapter 4: Making a Balanced and Nutritious Diet Plan

A healthy, well-balanced diet is essential for weight loss success. The key elements of a healthy eating strategy, how to determine your daily caloric needs, and advice for keeping a well-balanced diet are all covered in this chapter.

Knowledge of Macro nutrients

Carbohydrates, proteins, and fats are the three macro nutrients that the body needs in the greatest amounts.

1. Carbohydrates: The body gets its energy primarily from carbohydrates. Select complex carbohydrates over simple sugars and processed foods, such as whole grains, fruits, and vegetables.

2. Proteins: It's important to retain lean muscle mass when losing weight because it promotes muscle growth and repair. Choose lean sources of protein such as tofu, fish, poultry, and lentils.

3. Fats: Good fats are necessary for several biological processes. Limit saturated and trans fats found in fried and processed meals

while increasing sources of unsaturated fats such as avocados, almonds, and olive oil.

Determine Caloric Needs

A key step in developing a diet plan is figuring out how many calories you require each day. Estimates can be obtained using online calculators based on details like age, height, weight, degree of activity, and weight loss objectives.

Aim for a caloric deficit of between 500 and 750 calories each day to lose weight successfully. This method of losing weight gradually encourages long-term weight loss without depriving your body of the necessary nutrients.

Controlling portions and eating mindfully

Portion management techniques assist you to avoid overeating and let you indulge in a range of foods without consuming too many calories. To engage in mindful eating, pay attention to your body's signals of hunger and fullness while putting away all other distractions.

Planning and preparing meals

To ensure you always have wholesome options available, make your meals in advance. Meals prepared at home provide you control over the ingredients and serving amounts. Try out various cooking methods and recipes to keep your meals interesting and pleasurable.

Weight Loss and Hydration

Water consumption is crucial for weight loss. Water promotes digestion, regulates metabolism, and can lessen hunger sensations. Depending on your degree of activity and the weather, try to consume at least 8 cups of water each day.

The Function of Fiber

Whole grains, fruits, and vegetables are examples of foods high in fiber that add bulk to your diet and promote satiety. Additionally, they improve intestinal health and aid with digestion, which benefits general health.

Keeping away from Strict Diets

Although a calorie deficit is essential for weight loss, stay away from too-limiting diets that cut out entire food groups. The effective operation of your body and long-term success in keeping a healthy weight depends on balanced eating.

Conclusion

Developing a diet plan that is both balanced and nourishing is essential for weight loss. You can provide your body with the nutrition it needs to reach your goals by comprehending macro nutrients, figuring out your caloric needs, using portion management, and embracing mindful eating.

We'll move our attention to the significance of including exercise in your weight loss plan in Chapter 5. Keep in mind that maintaining consistency and changing your lifestyle to one that supports your well-being is crucial. Maintain your commitment, and success will come.

Chapter 5: The Function of Exercise in Weight Loss

A ny weight loss journey that is successful must include exercise. This chapter will cover the many advantages of physical activity, various weight-loss routines, and how to design a workout schedule that suits your preferences and goals.

The Advantages of Exercise for Losing Weight

In addition to helping you burn calories, exercise has several health advantages that can help you lose weight:

1. Increased Caloric Expenditure: Exercise burns calories, which, when combined with a balanced diet, results in a greater calorie deficit.

2. Preservation of Lean Muscle Mass: Muscle loss during weight loss is a possibility. Lean muscle mass preservation is aided by regular exercise, particularly resistance training, which is essential for a healthy metabolism.

3. Better Calorie Burning During Rest: Exercise can increase

your metabolism, resulting in more effective calorie burning even when you're at rest.

4. Improved Cardiovascular Health: Activities that increase cardiovascular fitness, such as jogging, swimming, or cycling, also increase stamina and endurance.

5. Mental Well-being: Exercising causes the production of endorphins, which lower stress, elevate mood, and improve general mental health.

6. Better Sleep: Regular exercise can enhance the quality of sleep, which is essential for slimming down and maintaining good health.

Exercises for Weight Loss: Types

Exercises that raise your heart rate and burn a lot of calories include 1. Cardiovascular exercises. Running, brisk walking, cycling, dancing, and aerobics are among the examples.

2. Strength training: Resistance training, whether done with weights or your body weight, helps maintain and grow muscle mass. This helps maintain a toned physique and a greater metabolic rate.

3. High-Intensity Interval Training (HIIT): HIIT involves switching back and forth between quick bursts of vigorous exercise and rest intervals. It is a quick technique to increase cardiovascular fitness and burn calories.

23

4. Exercises that increase flexibility and balance: Yoga and Pilates are great for enhancing flexibility, balance, and core strength, which can be used in conjunction with other routines.

Establishing a Workout Schedule

Consistency requires creating an exercise plan that fits your tastes and lifestyle:

1. Establish Realistic Goals: Clearly outline your fitness objectives for your weight loss goals. Start with moderate workouts, then progressively up the duration and intensity.

2. Plan Regular Workouts: Aim for 150 minutes or more of moderate-intensity activity per week, spread out over a few days.

3. Mix It Up: Include different exercises to keep your training interesting and prevent plateaus.

4. Listen to Your Body: Pay close attention to how exercise affects your body. To avoid injuries, give yourself enough time to relax and heal.

Continued Motivation

The secret to sticking with your fitness plan is to keep your motivation high:

1. Find a Workout Partner: Exercising with a friend or enrolling in a fitness class can be more fun and supportive of one another.

2. Track Your Progress: To keep track of your accomplishments and advancements, keep a workout notebook or utilize a fitness app.

3. Reward Yourself: As a means to maintain motivation, celebrate milestones and accomplishments of any size.

Conclusion

Exercise is essential to your weight loss efforts since it improves both your physical and emotional health. You will see good changes that support your overall success if you mix up your exercise regimen while remaining steadfast and motivated.

We will discuss the value of forming healthy habits in Chapter 6 to support your long-term weight loss objectives and lifestyle maintenance. Exercise is a celebration of what your body is capable of, not a punishment. The outcomes will come if you enthusiastically embrace the trip.

Chapter 6: Building Healthy Habits for Long-Term Success

Building healthy behaviors into your routine will help you lose weight in a sustainable way rather than just making short-term improvements. The significance of habits, techniques for developing them, and how they contribute to long-term success will all be covered in this chapter.

The Influence of Habit

Habits are instinctive behaviors that are developed via practice and repetition. You lay a solid basis for accomplishing and upholding your weight loss objectives by forming healthy habits.

Conscious Eating

Being fully present throughout meals, observing hunger and fullness cues, and appreciating each bite are all aspects of mindful eating. To avoid overeating and to enjoy your meal, learn to eat mindfully.

Typical Mealtimes

To establish a regulated eating routine, set regular mealtimes. Your metabolism may be regulated and impulsive eating can be avoided with regular meal timing.

Portion Regulation

By managing your portion sizes, you may indulge in your favorite foods while still sticking to your calorie budget. To encourage thoughtful portions, use smaller plates, provide reasonable servings, and refrain from eating directly from containers.

Prepare meals

To prevent impulsive, unhealthy decisions when hunger strikes, prepare healthful meals in advance. It is simpler to stick to your nutrition plan when you have pre-made meals or snacks on hand.

Discreet Snacking

To stave off hunger in between meals, choose nutrient-dense snacks like yogurt, fruits, veggies, almonds, or salad. Do not consume high-calorie, low-nutrient snacks since they may hinder your growth.

the routine of regular exercise

Consistently include exercise in your everyday regimen. To improve total fitness, aim for a balance of aerobic, strength, and flexibility exercises.

Active Way of Life

Whenever you can, include physical activity in your routine. Use the stairs rather than the elevator, go for a brief walk or ride a bike instead of driving, and look for opportunities to exercise throughout the day.

Proper Sleep

Make sleep a priority and strive for 7-9 hours of good sleep each night. A healthy sleep schedule benefits your overall well-being and aids in controlling hunger hormones.

Stress Reduction

Stress can cause emotional eating, which can interfere with your attempts to lose weight. Look for stress-reduction techniques that are healthful, such as yoga, deep breathing exercises, meditation, or time spent in nature.

Mercy for oneself and endurance

Throughout your weight-loss journey, be kind to yourself. Recognize that development may not always be straightforward and that setbacks are common. As you strive toward your goals, be patient and kind to yourself.

Responsibility and Assistance

Discuss your weight loss experience with a friend, a member of your family, or a support group. Sharing your struggles and achievements with someone else can motivate you and hold you accountable.

Conclusion

The secret to long-term success in weight loss and upholding a better lifestyle is to develop good habits. You may lay the groundwork for long-lasting positive change by including self-compassion, mindful eating, and regular exercise in your daily routine.

We will discuss emotional eating in Chapter 7 and how to stop doing it, giving you the tools you need to take charge of your relationship with food and emotions. Keep in mind that constant tiny steps result in big changes. Accept the process, and you'll see how it improves your life.

Chapter 7: Overcoming Emotional Eating

E motional eating is a frequent obstacle that lots of people run across when trying to lose weight. The origins of emotional eating, techniques for recognizing emotional triggers, and successful methods for overcoming this practice are all covered in this chapter.

Knowledge of Emotional Eating

Emotional eating is the practice of utilizing food as a coping method for feelings other than physical hunger, such as stress, melancholy, boredom, or anxiety. It frequently results in consuming unhealthy, high-calorie foods in large quantities, which can impede the process of losing weight.

Knowing Your Emotional Triggers

Breaking the pattern of emotional eating requires being able to identify emotional triggers. To keep note of your feelings and the circumstances in which you tend to turn to food, keep a journal. To better understand your triggers, look for patterns and recurring themes.

Engaging in Mindfulness

You can increase your awareness of your emotions and responses to them by practicing mindfulness. When you experience an emotional want to eat, pause and consider if you are indeed physically hungry or whether an emotional need is causing the impulse.

Adaptive coping techniques

Healthy coping strategies that handle your emotions without turning to food can take the place of emotional eating. Effective substitutes include:

1. Physical activity: To release endorphins and lower stress, engage in exercise or any other form of physical activity.

2. Journaling: To process emotions and find insight, write down your ideas and feelings.

3. Deep breathing and meditation: Use relaxation techniques to control stress and clear your mind.

4. Social Support: Discuss your feelings with a friend, a member of your family, or a therapist.

5. Hobbies and Activities: Take part in hobbies or enjoyable activities to occupy your time and block out emotional cravings.

Building a Support Network

Inform your network of friends, family, or a support group about your difficulties with emotional eating. You can stay on track and get rid of emotional eating tendencies by sharing your struggles and getting support.

Construction of Emotional Resilience

You can endure life's hardships without turning to food for consolation if you develop emotional resilience. Recognize that emotions are a normal part of life and use self-compassion when things are tough.

Conscious Eating Techniques

To stop emotional eating, incorporate mindful eating practices. Be sure to chew food carefully, enjoy each bite, and pay attention to your body's hunger and fullness signs.

Learning to Forgive

If you make a mistake and indulge in emotional eating, be kind to yourself. Keep in mind that it's a process and that failures present chances for learning and development. Be kind to yourself and get back on track without criticizing yourself.

Conclusion

A crucial first step to achieving successful and long-lasting weight loss is getting rid of emotional eating. You can escape the vicious cycle of emotional eating by becoming more aware of your emotional triggers, cultivating mindfulness, implementing healthy coping techniques, and getting support.

In Chapter 8, we'll discuss some obstacles and hurdles you can face when trying to lose weight and provide solutions. Keep in mind that you have the power to change the way you interact with food and emotions. Success will be within your grasp if you remain persistent.

Chapter 8: Overcoming Obstacles and Plateaus

A ny weight loss journey will inevitably have plateaus and obstacles. In this chapter, we'll look at the causes of plateaus, how to get through them, and how to persevere in the face of difficulties.

Recognizing Plateaus

A weight loss plateau is a time when, despite ongoing efforts, your weight remains unchanged. This is a typical occurrence as your body adjusts to changes in diet and exercise, which can be discouraging and demotivating.

the causes of plateaus

Weight loss plateaus can be caused by several things, including:

1. Metabolic Adaptation: As you lose weight, your metabolism can slow down, which would lower the amount of calories your body burns while at rest.

2. Muscle Gain: By including strength training in your regimen,

you may increase your lean muscle mass, which may counteract any fat loss.

3. Water Retention: Hormonal shifts and variations in sodium intake can temporarily increase water retention, which can conceal fat loss.

4. Lack of calorie Deficit: If your calorie intake is no longer producing a sizable deficit, weight loss may be coming to a halt.

Getting Over Plateaus

1. Reconsider Your Calorie Intake: Reassess your daily calorie requirements and modify your diet to produce a fresh deficit.

2. Change Your Exercise Routine: To prevent adaptation, switch up your workouts and give your body new exercises to adapt to.

3. Maintain Hydration: Drinking enough water can support your metabolism and aid in the removal of extra water weight.

4. Track Non-Scale Victories: Pay attention to non-scale achievements like improved fitness, more energy, or better-fitting apparel.

5. Exercise Consistency and Patience: Your body will eventually respond to your efforts with time because plateaus are transient.

overcoming obstacles

You can expect obstacles on your weight-loss journey. To

overcome obstacles, whether they be social gatherings, holidays, or stress, one must be tenacious and have a positive outlook.

1. Make a plan: Create a plan of action in advance to be ready for difficult circumstances. Bring healthful food to events or think of stress-relieving alternatives.

2. Exercise Moderation: Permit yourself to occasionally indulge, but be mindful of your portion sizes and your overall intake.

3. Focus on Progress, Not Perfection: Celebrate each step you take toward your goals while accepting the ups and downs as part of the process.

4. Learn from Setbacks: If you have setbacks, pinpoint the causes and create contingency plans to deal with similar circumstances in the future.

5. Seek Support: Rely on your support network when facing difficulties. Discussing your thoughts and feelings with someone else can be immensely beneficial.

Conclusion

Managing obstacles and plateaus is an essential component of the weight loss process. You can stay on track and keep moving toward your goals by comprehending the causes of plateaus and putting these solutions into practice.

We'll talk about the value of sleep for both weight loss and general health in Chapter 9. Keep in mind that every challenge you confront is a chance for development. If you stay dedicated, you'll come out stronger and closer to your goals.

Chapter 9: The Benefits of Sleep for Losing Weight

Sleep is essential for maintaining your general health and well-being, which includes controlling your weight. This chapter will cover the relationship between sleep and weight reduction, how sleep affects hormones and techniques for getting better sleep.

The Link Between Sleep and Weight Loss

The inability to lose weight and weight gain have both been linked to inadequate sleep. Lack of sleep can throw off your body's natural rhythms and impact the hormones that control your metabolism and hunger.

hormones and food cravings

Hormones that control hunger and satiety can become unbalanced as a result of sleep deprivation:

1. Ghrelin: Also referred to as the "hunger hormone," ghrelin levels rise during sleep deprivation, which increases appetite.

2. Leptin: Leptin is in charge of informing the brain when a person is full. Lack of sleep lowers leptin levels, which makes you feel more peckish and unsatisfied after meals.

3. Cortisol: Lack of sleep can raise cortisol levels, which can result in more stress and possible overeating, especially comfort foods with high-calorie counts.

Influence on Metabolism

Lack of sleep can affect your body's metabolism as well:

1. Lower Basal Metabolic Rate (BMR): Lack of sleep can cause your BMR, which measures how many calories your body burns while at rest, to drop.

2. Reduced Insulin Sensitivity: Lack of sleep may result in decreased insulin sensitivity, which may raise blood sugar levels and increase the risk of type 2 diabetes.

Techniques for Getting More Rest

Your efforts to lose weight can be favorably impacted by improving the quality of your sleep:

1. Create a Consistent Sleep Schedule: To balance your body's internal clock, go to bed and wake up at the same time every day, even on the weekends.

2. Create a Sleep-Friendly Environment: To encourage better sleep, make your bedroom cozy, quiet, and dark.

3. Limit Screen Time Before Bed: Blue light from screens and electronic gadgets might prevent the creation of melatonin, so avoid them at least an hour before bed.

4. Practice Relaxation Techniques: Before going to bed, relax your body and mind by reading, doing some meditation, or having a warm bath.

5. Limit Caffeine and Alcohol Consumption: Limit caffeine and alcohol intake because they might interfere with sleep cycles, especially in the evening.

6. Exercise During the Day: Regular exercise can enhance the quality of your sleep, but you should avoid doing an intensive workout right before bed.

Sleep as a Priority for Successful Weight Loss

Recognize that getting enough sleep is crucial to your efforts to lose weight. To support your general health and weight loss goals, aim for 7-9 hours of good sleep each night.

Conclusion

The ability to sleep properly is essential for both weight loss and general well-being. You may maximize your weight loss efforts and achieve long-term success by comprehending the relationship between sleep, hormones, and metabolism and putting measures for better sleep into practice.

In Chapter 10, we'll look at how stress affects weight loss and give you practical stress-reduction strategies to help you on your way. Remember that a well-rested body is better able to overcome obstacles, maintain motivation, and arrive at your goal.

Chapter 10: Weight Loss and Stress Management

S tress has a big impact on your ability to lose weight since it alters your hormone levels, eating patterns, and general health. This chapter will examine the link between stress and weight gain, practical stress reduction methods, and how to keep your equilibrium under trying circumstances.

Stress and Weight Gain

Chronic stress sets off several physiological reactions that might contribute to weight gain and make it more difficult to lose weight:

1. powerful desires: As a coping mechanism for emotions, stress can cause powerful desires, especially for comfort foods high in calories.

2. Cortisol Release: The body releases cortisol when under stress, which can cause fat to accumulate, particularly in the abdomen region.

3. Disrupted Eating Patterns: Stress can result in erratic eating habits, which can cause overeating or meal skipping.

4. Emotional Eating: Stress can lead to emotional eating, in which hunger is replaced by using food as a coping method to deal with emotions.

Techniques for Effective Stress Management

Maintaining a healthy lifestyle and achieving your weight loss objectives depend on appropriate stress management:

1. Exercise: Get regular exercise to release endorphins, which are effective stress relievers in nature.

2. Mindfulness and Meditation: To relieve stress and enhance emotional well-being, practice mindfulness and meditation practices.

3. Deep breathing exercises: Deep breathing exercises have been shown to lower stress levels and soothe the neurological system.

4. Time management: To lower stress, prioritize chores, establish attainable goals, and refrain from over committing oneself.

5. Creative Outlets: As a way to express and let go of feelings, partake in creative endeavors like writing, painting, or music-making.

6. Disconnect from Technology: To relieve tension and sharpen

43

focus, take pauses from using electronics.

Maintaining Balance During Difficulties

There are many problems in life, thus it's important to maintain balance to avoid stress-related weight gain:

1. Develop Self-Compassion: Avoid self-criticism and be kind to yourself when going through difficult times.

2. Continue with Healthy Routines: Maintain your healthy diet and exercise routines, since they can offer stability and control during stressful situations.

3. Seek Support: In difficult circumstances, turn to your support network for advice and inspiration.

4. Keep an eye on the big picture: Keep in mind your long-term objectives and that difficulties are just temporary obstacles.

5. Adapt and Adjust: Maintain a flexible attitude and be willing to modify your weight loss strategy as necessary without becoming disheartened.

Conclusion

Effective stress management is essential for keeping a healthy weight and general well-being. You can successfully deal with pressures and maintain your weight reduction journey by using stress management techniques and maintaining balance during trying moments.

We will discuss mindful eating and how it affects weight reduction and your relationship with food in Chapter 11. Keep in mind that stress is a natural part of life, but how you handle it will affect how your journey turns out. Remain strong, and success will come.

Chapter 11: Embracing Mindful Eating

A powerful technique called mindful eating can change how you feel about food and help you reach your weight loss objectives. In this chapter, we will examine the idea of mindful eating, as well as its advantages and doable implementation methods.

How Does Mindful Eating Work?

The practice of mindful eating involves being completely present and nonjudgmental as you eat. It entails focusing on the flavor, feel, and aroma of food as well as picking up on hunger and fullness cues.

The Advantages of Mindful Consumption

Adopting mindful eating can have a variety of positive effects on your physical and mental health, including:

1. Improved Digestion: As you chew food completely and

give your body time to properly absorb it, mindful eating encourages improved digestion.

2. Managed Portion Sizes: You may avoid overeating by paying attention to your hunger and fullness cues. This will help you eat until you are satisfied.

3. Increased Satisfaction: You can enjoy your meals more and feel fuller by taking your time with each bite.

4. Less Emotional Eating: By learning to discern between physical hunger and emotional cravings, mindful eating can help you control your tendency to overeat when you're under stress or feeling upset.

5. Weight Management: Mindful eating techniques can aid in weight loss and support the maintenance of a healthy weight.

How to Practice Mindful Eating

1. Eat Without Distractions: Steer clear of watching television or conducting other things while you eat. Concentrate just on your meal.

2. Chew thoroughly and slowly, savoring the flavors and textures of your food.

3. Take a Breath Between Bites: Put down your fork or knife between bites and pause to assess your appetite and fullness.

4. Use Your Senses: Be aware of the way your food looks, smells, and tastes.

5. Recognize Emotional Triggers: Check to see whether you're eating out of emotion rather than actual hunger.

6. Consume Food Regularly: Create a regular eating schedule to avoid acute hunger, which can result in overeating.

Improving One's Relationship with Food

You can have a healthy and balanced relationship with food by practicing mindful eating:

1. Avoid Food Guilt: Let go of guilt and criticism related to dietary decisions. A balanced eating strategy includes occasionally allowing oneself to indulge without feeling bad.

2. Be Kind to Yourself: Exercise self-compassion and refrain from critical thoughts about your eating habits.

3. Pay Attention to Your Body: Pay attention to your body's indications of hunger and fullness.

4. Celebrate Food Diversity: To have a well-rounded dining experience, embrace a wide range of foods and cuisines.

Conclusion

Adopting mindful eating can completely change your approach to weight loss and your relationship with food in general. You may develop a healthier and more mindful approach to feeding your body by practicing awareness, enjoying every bite, and cultivating a good attitude about food.

In Chapter 12, we'll talk about the importance of social support for weight loss and how creating a solid support system can help you succeed. A lifetime practice that nourishes both your body and soul, mindful eating is not a diet. Your path will be filled with growth and positive changes if you remain present and committed.

Chapter 12: Utilizing the Influence of Social Support

Having social support can be quite helpful while trying to lose weight. In this chapter, we'll look at the importance of social support, how it can increase your drive and dedication, and how to create a solid support system.

The Vitality of Social Support

Starting a weight loss journey can be difficult, but having a support network can be very helpful. Social assistance offers:

1. Words of encouragement from friends, family, or support networks can serve as a positive reinforcement of your accomplishments and abilities.

2. Accountability: Staying on track might be made easier when you are aware that others are aware of your goals.

3. Compassion: Those in your network of support might feel your struggles and show compassion when things get tough.

4. Shared Experiences: Making connections with those traveling

a similar path might provide insightful advice and success hacks.

Increasing Your Support System

Here are some methods for creating a powerful support system:

1. Communicate Your Goals: Tell trusted family members or friends about your plans to reduce weight and why they are important to you.

2. Join Support Groups: Look for neighborhood or online forums for people who are going through the same thing.

3. Find a Workout Partner: Team up with someone who can exercise with you regularly and shares your interests in fitness.

4. Seek Professional Support: Think about meeting with a counselor or weight reduction coach who can offer knowledgeable direction and inspiration.

5. Be Strict: Avoid individuals who might undermine your efforts and surround yourself with those who are encouraging and upbeat about your ambitions.

How to Deal with Unwanted Advice

Social support is helpful, but you could also get unwanted criticism or advice. Here's how to respond:

1. Maintain your confidence: Irrespective of what others may think, believe in your development and ambitions.

51

2. Inform Others: Explain the rationale behind your decisions and inform others of your journey.

3. Establish Boundaries: Politely but forcefully establish boundaries with individuals who provide unwelcome criticism or advice.

4. Concentrate on the Positive: Surround yourself with people who encourage you and offer helpful assistance.

Being an encouraging presence

As you accept assistance, keep in mind to give back and encourage others on their journeys:

1. Encourage your network: congratulate them on their accomplishments and offer assistance when things go tough.

2. Actively Listen: Show empathy and compassion when people are sharing their stories.

3. Share Knowledge: While respecting individual differences, provide practical advice and insights based on your experiences.

Conclusion

Social support is an important tool that can increase your motivation and fortitude as you embark on a weight loss journey. You can develop a community of support and understanding by creating a strong support network and being a supportive influence in return. This will help you move closer to your goals.

We'll look at methods for overcoming obstacles and maintaining motivation throughout your weight loss journey in Chapter 13. Remember that you are not walking this route alone. Accept the strength of social support, and together you may affect astonishing changes.

Chapter 13: Recovering from Failure and Maintaining Motivation

Any journey to lose weight will inevitably experience setbacks, but how you respond to them will have a big impact on your success. This chapter will cover typical obstacles and setbacks, solutions for them, and methods for maintaining motivation along the road.

Recognizing setbacks

There are many different types of setbacks, including weight plateaus, emotional eating episodes, and missed workouts. It's crucial to see setbacks as chances for growth and learning rather than failures.

Techniques for Overcoming Obstacles

1. Develop Self-Compassion: Avoid self-criticism when you experience disappointments and be kind to yourself. Remind yourself that everyone has obstacles along the way.

2. Examine the Trigger: Determine what led to the failure, such as emotional stress, a lack of planning, or outside influences.

You can create tactics to avoid similar setbacks in the future by understanding the cause.

3. Reevaluate Your Goals: Remind yourself of your long-term objectives and the motivations behind your initial weight loss efforts. Make use of them as inspiration to get back on course.

4. Focus on Progress, Not Perfection: Despite setbacks, celebrate each modest success and constructive improvement. Realize that development is not necessarily a linear process.

5. Have Realistic Expectations: Recognize that losing weight requires patience and perseverance. To avoid feeling overwhelmed, set goals that are both attainable and reasonable.

Keeping the Motivation

It can be difficult to stay motivated while traveling, but the following techniques can help:

1. Visualize Success: Envision achieving your weight-loss objectives and enjoying the advantages of a healthier lifestyle.

2. Use positive affirmations: Repeating positive affirmations regularly will help you stay confident and upbeat.

3. Monitor Your Progress: Log your accomplishments, adjustments, and landmarks in a journal or with a monitoring app.

4. Reward Yourself: Give yourself non-food prizes like a spa day or new workout clothing to acknowledge your successes, no

matter how minor.

5. Find Inspiration: To stay motivated, read success stories, follow fitness influencers, and surround oneself with inspirational material.

6. Modify Your Approach: If you find yourself lacking enthusiasm, think about experimenting with different exercises, dishes, or strategies to keep things interesting.

Developing Resistance

Resilience is the capacity to overcome obstacles and failures. Increase resiliency by:

1. Developing Coping Strategies: To handle stress, find healthy coping strategies like meditation, hobbies, or chatting with friends.

2. Seeking assistance: For assistance and understanding through trying times, turn to your support network.

3. Embracing Flexibility: Recognize that failures are inevitable along the way, and be prepared to modify your strategy as necessary.

Conclusion

A successful weight loss journey requires overcoming obstacles and maintaining motivation. You can overcome obstacles and proceed with your goals by developing self-compassion, learning from failures, and keeping a positive mindset.

We will look at methods for sustaining weight loss and developing a long-term, healthy lifestyle in Chapter 14. Recall that on this transforming road, motivation and resilience go hand in hand. You will attain extraordinary outcomes if you remain committed.

Chapter 14: Sustaining Weight Loss for Life

L
ong-term success depends on maintaining weight loss and adopting a healthy lifestyle. This chapter will cover methods for maintaining weight loss, forming healthy routines, and developing a well-rounded outlook on health and well-being.

The Value of Sustainable Behavior

While reaching weight reduction objectives is admirable, keeping the results is just as important. Sustainable behaviors lay the groundwork for long-term success.

Consider your general health

Turn your attention away from weight loss and toward your general health and well-being. For energy and vitality, emphasize feeding your body with nutrient-dense foods and participating in frequent physical activity.

Keep eating mindfully

Even after you've met your weight loss objectives, keep up your attentive eating habits. Savoring each meal and eating mindfully can promote a healthy relationship with food, avoid weight gain, and keep it off.

Make physical activity a habit

Instead of seeing exercise as a means to an end, consider it a necessary component of your daily routine. Find physical things you like to do and incorporate them into your daily life.

Accept Variety

Adopt a flexible approach to food and avoid rigid diets. Embrace a wide variety of nutrient-dense foods, such as fresh produce, whole grains, lean meats, and healthy fats.

New Objectives

Set new objectives once you've met your initial weight reduction targets to continue growing and challenging yourself. These objectives may be on health, such as lowering stress, or they may be fitness-related, like running a 5K.

Track Your Development

Keep a record of your fitness and health accomplishments to stay inspired and spot any problems early on.

Prepare for difficulties

Recognize that obstacles will come your way and that it's okay to experience failure occasionally. Maintain your adaptability and be ready to go through challenging times.

Put self-care first

Take care of your mental and emotional health. To control stress and preserve a good mindset, engage in self-care.

Seek Assistance

Keep looking to your support system for inspiration and motivation. Be in the company of inspiring people who will elevate your spirit.

Honor Your Success

Celebrate both achieving your weight loss objectives and your dedication to leading a healthier lifestyle. Be proud of your accomplishments and the work you put into your path.

Conclusion

The key to maintaining weight loss is forming healthy habits that you can follow for the rest of your life. You can attain long-lasting success by putting an emphasis on overall health, maintaining a mindful diet and exercise, setting new goals, and placing a high priority on self-care.

We will review your transformational journey, praise your development, and provide some parting words of wisdom in the final chapter, Chapter 15. Keep in mind that this is a voyage of personal growth. Your healthy and fulfilling life is waiting for you if you remain committed.

Chapter 15: A Transformational Journey

I'm happy to hear that you've succeeded in your weight loss goals! This chapter honors your metamorphosis and looks back on the outstanding strides you've achieved. Keep in mind that this journey is about the experiences and growth you have along the road as you start the next chapter of your life.

Thinking Back on Your Successes

Think back on your progress for a moment. Celebrate all of your accomplishments, no matter how big or small, and give credit to your hard work and perseverance.

Accepting a New Way of Life

Your journey to losing weight has likely resulted in substantial lifestyle adjustments. Make these beneficial changes a permanent part of your life by accepting them.

Developing Gratitude

Thank your loved ones for their support, for the difficulties that helped you get stronger, and for the learning opportunities.

The Influence of Self-Reflection

You've probably discovered more about yourself on this adventure than you ever thought possible. Accept the journey of self-discovery and keep developing.

Posing New Objectives

It's time to set new objectives now that one adventure is over. What further goals do you have? Remember that you can attain your goals, whether they are focused on your health, profession, or personal development.

Supporting Others

As you rejoice in your accomplishments, think about how you may motivate and encourage others as they travel their paths. Your expertise and knowledge may influence the course of another person's life.

Acknowledging Imperfection

Keep in mind that perfection is not the objective. Accept your flaws because they make you special. Maintain your progress-oriented mindset while growing and improving.

Upholding Self-Care

Prioritize your well-being and self-care as you go forward. It's crucial to look after your needs if you want to live a healthy and satisfying life.

Taking Pride in Your Transformation

Celebrate your personal growth. You have accomplished something quite remarkable, and you should be pleased with yourself.

Final Messages of Inspiration

Keep in mind that this adventure is still ongoing and has no beginning or end. Take in every second, value every encounter, and keep working toward happiness and improvement.

Conclusion

Your quest to lose weight involves a significant internal transformation as well as outward bodily changes. Accept the knowledge you have gained, the difficulties you have faced, and the person you have evolved into.

Carry the self-assurance, fortitude, and tenacity that got you this far into the future. You can control your fate and design a life that is healthy, fulfilling, and happy.

Once more, congratulations on your transformational path. There are countless options, and the future is promising. You will continue to succeed if you welcome it with open arms.

II

The Power of Intermittent Fasting

*"Unlock your body's potential and discover the power
of intermittent fasting. With this transformative
journey, you can tap into your body's resilience and
vitality. Embrace the discipline of intermittent fasting
and unlock a healthier, more vibrant you.
Intermittent fasting is a journey of self-control that
leads to extraordinary results."*

Introduction

Welcome to "The Power of Intermittent Fasting," a thorough introduction to one of the most effective and thoroughly researched ways to enhance your general health and well-being. In this part, we'll look at the amazing advantages of intermittent fasting and how it can improve a variety of elements of your life, including longevity, mental acuity, and weight management.

It has been practiced by numerous civilizations and religions throughout human history for a variety of reasons; intermittent fasting is not a new trend. On the other hand, tremendous physiological and psychological effects of this eating pattern have just come to light thanks to scientific studies.

This part tries to clear up any myths or misunderstandings you may have about intermittent fasting and give you a thorough grasp of it. We will explore the scientific underpinnings of how intermittent fasting impacts our bodies, outlining the complex pathways that result in enhanced fat burning, enhanced brain function, and higher energy.

Furthermore, "The Power of Intermittent Fasting" will walk

you through how to apply intermittent fasting to your everyday life practically. This book has something for everyone, whether you're a beginner looking to get started or an expert seeking advanced tactics.

You will be given the information and resources required to maximize your success with intermittent fasting in each chapter. You will learn how to customize intermittent fasting to your lifestyle and goals, covering everything from different fasting techniques to meal planning and exercise integration.

To give you a strong basis for the following chapters, let's first discuss the background and history of intermittent fasting before getting into the specifics. Use this book as your go-to guide to maximizing the benefits of intermittent fasting and transforming your health and well-being.

Chapter 16: The History of Intermittent Fasting

Despite being popular in contemporary wellness circles, intermittent fasting is not a brand-new idea. Long before the development of agriculture and the practicality of a three-meal-a-day schedule, throughout the history of humanity, our predecessors engaged in intermittent fasting out of necessity.

Food was limited in the past, and our hunter-gatherer forefathers experienced periods of abundance and scarcity. Because the availability of food determined their eating habits, they evolved the capacity to perform at their best while fasting.

In addition to being a part of human history, these fasting periods were also a significant component of many cultural and religious traditions. Fasting was used to cultivate self-control, spiritual purity, and a closer relationship with the divine.

Intermittent fasting has had a significant impact on history, even more recent history. Plato, Aristotle, and Benjamin Franklin were just a few of the thinkers and historical luminaries who supported fasting for its possible mental clarity and health benefits.

The practice of intermittent fasting was gradually undermined by the development of modern agriculture and the abundance of food. Our eating habits altered as a result of easy access to food, which fueled an increase in constant nibbling and excessive calorie consumption.

However, as knowledge of human physiology and nutrition increased, researchers started to look again at the idea of intermittent fasting and discovered its extraordinary effects on the body and mind. Numerous scientific research conducted over the past few decades have supported the premise that intermittent fasting can be an effective strategy for enhancing health and well-being.

We will examine the science behind intermittent fasting and how it can be used to maximize the potential of your body and mind in the chapters that follow. Let's explore the background and roots of intermittent fasting to better understand how this age-old practice might transform the way we think about nutrition and wellness.

Chapter 17: Understanding the Science of Intermittent Fasting

We must go into the scientific theories that support this revolutionary eating strategy to properly understand the potential of intermittent fasting. Intermittent fasting affects several subtle physiological mechanisms that power its positive benefits in our well-honed biological machines.

Autophagy and cellular repair

The effects of intermittent fasting on cellular repair and autophagy are among its most amazing features. When we are fasting, when our bodies are not digesting food, they turn their attention to cellular upkeep and repair. Our cells naturally remove damaged parts and recycle them to support cellular health through a process called autophagy.

Cells can get rid of accumulated trash and malfunctioning organelles by engaging in autophagy. This procedure increases cellular longevity and efficiency, which promotes general health and longevity. According to studies, intermittent fasting can increase autophagy, which enhances cellular resilience and function.

Controlling blood sugar levels with insulin

Also significantly affecting insulin sensitivity and blood sugar control is intermittent fasting. Our insulin levels fall when we are fasting, making our cells more responsive to the hormone. By regulating blood sugar levels, this improved sensitivity lowers the likelihood of insulin resistance and type 2 diabetes.

Individuals with insulin resistance may see improvements in their health and less need for medication by implementing intermittent fasting. This fasting strategy also promotes the body to use fat storage as a source of energy, which helps with weight loss and metabolic health.

hormonal control

Intermittent fasting has a significant impact on several hormones in our bodies. For instance, growth hormone increases during periods of fasting, promoting fat burning, muscle growth, and tissue regeneration. Fasting is also associated with higher levels of norepinephrine, a hormone that promotes fat breakdown and benefits weight loss.

The production of brain-derived neurotrophic factor (BDNF), a protein that supports brain health and cognitive function, can also be positively impacted by intermittent fasting. The brain's capacity to adapt and make new connections, known as neuroplasticity, which improves memory and learning, is greatly influenced by BDNF.

Enhanced Weight Loss and Fat Burning

Weight loss is a major driver behind the adoption of intermittent fasting for many people. Through several factors, such as enhanced fat burning, decreased calorie intake, and better metabolism, intermittent fasting promotes weight loss.

The body switches to fat as its main energy source when fasting since it uses up its glycogen reserves. This metabolic change speeds up the burning of fat and aids in weight loss, especially when accompanied by a healthy diet and regular exercise.

Reduced Inflammation

Numerous health problems, such as cardiovascular disease, autoimmune diseases, and even some malignancies, are associated with chronic inflammation. By blocking proinflammatory signals and encouraging the creation of anti-inflammatory molecules, intermittent fasting has been demonstrated to help lower inflammation in the body.

Intermittent fasting can promote general health, lower the chance of developing chronic diseases, and promote a longer, healthier life by reducing inflammation.

Finally, the research on intermittent fasting reveals a wide range of health advantages for our bodies and minds. Intermittent fasting offers a comprehensive strategy for enhancing health and well-being, from hormonal management and hormone-related processes like autophagy and cellular repair to accelerated fat burning. In the next chapters, we'll discuss different

73

types of intermittent fasting and how you can incorporate this effective technique into your lifestyle for the best outcomes.

Chapter 18: Starting Intermittent Fasting

T hanks for starting the process of accepting the benefits of intermittent fasting! Now that you have a basic understanding of the science underlying this revolutionary method, it's time to start your journey with intermittent fasting. We will walk you through the necessary procedures to begin intermittent fasting in this chapter, preparing you for success.

1. Speak with a Medical Professional

It's important to speak with a healthcare provider before beginning any new dietary or lifestyle practices, especially if you have any current medical ailments or worries. While many people find intermittent fasting to be safe and healthy, it might not be appropriate for everyone. A licensed healthcare professional can evaluate your unique medical requirements and provide tailored advice.

2. Select the Proper Fasting Technique

You can choose an intermittent fasting approach that suits your lifestyle and preferences from a variety of available options. Popular regimens for fasting include:

The 16/8 approach entails an 8-hour window of eating followed by 16 hours of fasting each day. It's one of the easiest methods and is simple to incorporate into daily life.

The 5:2 Diet: Using this strategy, you eat normally five days a week while cutting back to about 500–600 calories on the other two days that aren't consecutive.

Eat-Stop-Eat: This technique entails going without food once or twice every week for a full 24 hours.

Alternate-Day Fasting: As the name implies, you alternate between days when you fast and days when you normally eat.

Warrior Diet: This strategy calls for skipping meals during the day and having a substantial dinner.

You can experiment with several fasting techniques to find the one that works best for you because each one has its special advantages.

3. Start slowly.

It's a good idea to ease into intermittent fasting if you're new to it. Increase the interval between your final meal of the day and your first meal the next day to start. Try moving your breakfast, for instance, if you typically have it from 8 AM to 10 AM or 11 AM. Your body will have time to acclimate to the fasting period thanks to this gradual change.

4. Keep hydrated.

Maintaining hydration is crucial when fasting. Generally speaking, during fasting periods, water, herbal teas, and black coffee are allowed and can help reduce hunger. Drinking enough water helps the body's natural detoxifying processes.

5. Always Eat Balanced Meals

Even though intermittent fasting does not specify particular meals, it is crucial to keep up a nutritious and balanced diet within your eating window. Emphasize full, nutrient-dense foods, such as fresh produce, lean meats and fish, healthy fats, and whole grains. Avoid consuming processed and sugary foods in excess because they can impede your progress and jeopardize your health.

6. Observe your body.

Finding what works best for your body and way of life is what intermittent fasting is all about—not following rigid rules. Pay close attention to how you feel while eating and fasting. Consider changing your fasting strategy or attempting a different one if one leaves you feeling extremely worn out or agitated.

7. Be dependable

To reap the full benefits of intermittent fasting, consistency is essential. Be as consistent with your fasting regimen as you can, but also give yourself some leeway and forgiveness. Because life can be unpredictable, it's acceptable to occasionally change your plans.

As you begin your intermittent fasting adventure, keep in mind that you are learning about yourself and working to improve yourself. With patience and an open mind, embrace the trip, and you'll probably notice improvements in your overall well-being, mental clarity, and physical health.

The 30-Day Intermittent Fasting Schedule in Brief

Week One: The 16/8 Approach

1. Day 1: Setting goals, learning the 16/8 approach, and preparing your meals.

2. Day 2: Gradual Adjustment: Gradually extend your window of fasting and shorten your eating window.

3. Day 3: Hydration and Nutrition: Maintaining hydration and making sure you're getting a balanced diet when you eat.

4. Building Resilience Day 4: Managing Hunger Cravings and Finding Alternatives to Suppress Appetite.

5. Day 5: Fasting and Exercise: For greater benefits, incorporate light exercise into fasting intervals.

6. Managing social engagements and gatherings while fasting on Day 6: Social Challenges.

7. Day 7 - Weekly Review: Evaluate your development, make modifications, and recognize minor successes.

The 5:2 Method in Week 2

1. *Day 8 - Introduction to 5:2: Recognizing the advantages of the 5:2 approach.*

2. *Day 9 - The Two Fasting Days: Meal planning for your two separate fasting days.*

3. *On days when you aren't fasting, you should concentrate on eating nourishing foods.*

4. *On Day 11, focus on mindful eating to prevent overindulgence.*

5. *Day 12: Hunger Management: Successful methods for overcoming hunger on days when you're fasting.*

6. *Day 13: Exercise regimen: Create an exercise regimen that goes along with your fasting schedule.*

7. *Day 14 - Weekly Check-In: Evaluate your development and make the required corrections.*

The Eat-Stop-Eat Method in Week Three

1. *Day 15 - Overview of Eat-Stop-Eat: Getting to know the 24-hour fasting strategy.*

2. *Day 16 - Getting Ready for a 24-Hour Fast: Increasing Your Fasting Period Gradually.*

3. *Day 17: The Fasting Day: Maintaining activity and concentration throughout the 24-hour fast.*

4. *Day 18: Breaking the Fast: Make healthy food selections to break your fast successfully.*

5. *Day 19: Hydration and Detoxification: The function of water during fasting and its benefits for detoxification.*

6. *Day 20 - Using Fasting and Exercise Together to Get the Most Out of Your Fast.*

7. *Day 21: Weekly Reflection: Examining your development and maintaining motivation.*

Finding Your Balance in Week Four

1. *Transitioning from a rigid fast to intuitive eating on Day 22.*

2. *Day 23: Understanding hunger and satiety signs by listening to your body.*

3. *Day 24: Understanding the connection between the mind and body and fasting.*

4. *The effects of stress and sleep on intermittent fasting are discussed on day 25, "Sleep and Stress."*

5. *Day 26: Marking Progress: Honoring your victories and anniversaries.*

6. *Day 27: Handling Reversals: Managing Occasional Slip-Ups and Regaining Focus.*

7. *Planning for the final week of the 30-day journey begins on day 28.*

Week 5: Maintaining the Way of Life

1. *Day 29: Making intermittent fasting a permanent way of life after the 30-day challenge.*

2. *Day 30: Celebrating Your Transformation and Progress and Looking Back on Your Journey.*

3. *A Journey to Better Health: A Summary of the Influence and Benefits of Intermittent Fasting.*

FREQUENTLY ASKED QUESTIONS or FAQs

Can I drink water while I'm fasting?

Yes, it's important to stay hydrated during fasting. Black

coffee, herbal teas, and water are permitted.

Does intermittent fasting cause muscular wasting?

Intermittent fasting shouldn't cause muscle loss when done properly. Maintaining muscular mass requires both a protein-rich diet and regular exercise.

Q3: Can I work out when I'm fasting?

Yes, for further benefits, light to moderate exercise is advised during fasting periods.

Is intermittent fasting appropriate for all people?

For people with eating problems, those who are pregnant or nursing, or those who have specific medical concerns, intermittent fasting may not be a good idea. Before beginning, you must speak with a medical expert.

Can I include intermittent fasting in other diets?

Yes, for better outcomes, intermittent fasting can be paired with different healthy diets like the Mediterranean or ketogenic diet.

Q6: Can intermittent fasting aid in enhancing cognitive performance?

Yes, research indicates that intermittent fasting may benefit brain health. The protein brain-derived neurotrophic factor (BDNF), which maintains brain function and may lower the risk of neurodegenerative disorders, is produced more readily when people fast.

What may I eat when there are designated eating windows?

Focus on eating nutrient-dense foods including fruits, vegetables, whole grains, lean proteins, and healthy fats during the meal windows. To maximize the health benefits, stay away from processed and sugary foods.

A8: Can there be unfavorable side effects from intermittent fasting?

When first adjusting to intermittent fasting, some people may experience negative side effects like irritation, exhaustion, or dizziness. However, when the body becomes used to the fasting schedule, these symptoms are frequently transient and tend to get better.

Q9: Can I have wine while fasting?

Alcohol should be avoided throughout the fasting period because it can disrupt the fast and cause dehydration. If you decide to consume alcohol, do it moderately and throughout your meal window.

How can I keep up my fasting schedule while traveling?

Your fasting schedule may be hampered by travel, but with some preparation, you can maintain it. Be prepared with wholesome snacks, arrange your eating and fasting times in advance, and be adaptable to changing your schedule to fit your travel plans.

Certainly! Let's go on to the following section:

How to Travel Successfully While Intermittent Fasting

Even while the 30-day intermittent fasting plan is a great method to get started on your trip, it's crucial to include the following critical advice to make it even more successful and enjoyable:

1. When it's time to eat, concentrate on eating balanced meals that contain a variety of nutrients. This will give you energy and satisfaction all day long.

2. Pay attention to your body's messages by keeping an ear to the ground. It's acceptable to modify your fasting schedule or seek advice from a healthcare provider if you feel ill or overly exhausted.

3. Plan Your Meals: Making pre-planned meals can help you stay on track with your fasting schedule and prevent impulsive or harmful food decisions.

4. Practice Mindful Eating: During your eating windows, pay attention and be mindful. This can assist you in appreciating your meals more and in identifying your body's signals of hunger and fullness.

5. Get Enough Sleep: Sleep is crucial for your body's healing and general well-being. Make sure you receive enough sleep to support your journey with intermittent fasting.

6. Stay Active: Include regular exercise in your daily routine.

Intermittent fasting can enhance the benefits of exercise, which will improve your general health.

7. Track Your Progress: Use apps or a journal to record your progress and acknowledge your successes. Observing your progress helps keep you inspired.

8. Be patient because every person's results may be different. Be kind to yourself and have faith in the process. Consistency is essential and takes time for lasting results.

Conclusion

Congratulations! The beginner's 30-day intermittent fasting journey is over. You've built a strong foundation for a healthier lifestyle by following this step-by-step manual and adopting the crucial advice. More than just a fad, intermittent fasting is a potent tool that can alter your relationship with food and enhance your general well-being.

Always keep in mind that everyone's journey is different, making it crucial to choose an intermittent fasting strategy that complements your lifestyle and interests. Whether you go with the 16/8, 5:2, or Eat-Stop-Eat approach, the most important thing is to follow it consistently and with awareness.

Be accepting of the changes taking place in your body and mind as you continue on your intermittent fasting journey. Celebrate each accomplishment, no matter how minor, and view failures as teaching moments. You're well on your way to enjoying the lasting advantages of intermittent fasting; this is a lifelong process.

The metabolic health, general well-being, and weight management can all significantly improve after a 30-day intermittent fasting excursion. Always pay attention to your body, maintain consistency, and ask for help if you need it. Intermittent fasting can develop into a sustaining and fulfilling lifestyle choice with commitment and mindfulness. Why then wait? Start today on the revolutionary path to greater health!

A flexible and accessible approach to well-being, intermittent fasting offers a variety of techniques to meet personal preferences. It's crucial to speak with a healthcare provider before beginning any lifestyle change, especially if you have any underlying medical issues. To become a healthier and happier version of yourself, stay dedicated, practice patience, and reap the many advantages of intermittent fasting. Cheers to a successful and rewarding 30-day experiment in intermittent fasting!

Chapter 19: Which Type of Intermittent Fasting Is Right for You

I t's time to investigate the many available fasting regimens now that you've decided to adopt intermittent fasting. Each technique caters to various lifestyles and interests while offering special advantages and flexibility. We will go deeper into the most common forms of intermittent fasting in this chapter to help you decide which one best suits your objectives and daily schedule.

1. **16/8 Approach**

The Leangains protocol, sometimes referred to as the 16/8 method, is one of the most straightforward and well-liked methods of intermittent fasting. It entails reducing your eating window to 8 hours and fasting for 16 hours each day. You might eat between 12 PM and 8 PM one day and then fast between 8 PM and 12 PM the next.

Given that it enables you to skip breakfast and begin eating later in the day, this strategy is simple to adopt into a regular daily schedule. Many people believe that the 16/8 technique strikes a fair compromise between the advantages of fasting and its usefulness.

2. 5:2 Approach

In the 5:2 diet, you consume your regular diet for five days a week while limiting your calorie intake to 500–600 calories on the other two days that are not consecutive. Choosing nutrient-dense foods on fasting days is crucial to ensuring that you still get the necessary vitamins and minerals.

The calorie restriction on fasting days makes this strategy more difficult for certain people. However, it allows for the freedom to select which days to fast, making it flexible to a range of schedules.

3. Eat-Stop-Eat

The Eat-Stop-Eat approach calls for fasting once or twice every week for a complete 24 hours. For instance, you might finish your meal at 7 PM one day and wait until 7 PM the next day to eat again.

Although it may seem difficult, this approach enables a total reset of the body's metabolic functions. During fasting time, it's crucial to stay hydrated and break the fast with a healthy meal.

4. Day-by-Day Fasting

You alternate between fasting days and days when you eat normally when you practice alternate-day fasting. In contrast to days when you aren't fasting, when you are eating normally, you may ingest relatively few calories.

This approach might not be ideal for everyone because some people could find it difficult to keep up with severe fasting days. However, it can be a successful strategy to encourage weight loss and metabolic flexibility for individuals who can stick with the program.

5. Battle Diet

On the Warrior Diet, you eat one substantial meal at night and fast during the day. Small portions of raw fruits, vegetables, and lean protein sources are permitted during the fasting period.

People who find it easier to fast throughout the day and prefer a larger meal in the evening would find this strategy appealing. It promotes a more instinctual feeding style that is consistent with the theory of how ancient warriors may have eaten.

6. Customized Method

In addition to the techniques already discussed, intermittent fasting can be tailored to meet your specific requirements. To create a plan that fits your lifestyle and goals, you can experiment with fasting lengths, eating windows, and frequency.

Always keep in mind that selecting an intermittent fasting strategy you can stick with over the long run is the key to success. For the benefits of intermittent fasting to fully manifest, flexibility and consistency are essential.

Be mindful that different people may react differently as you experiment with various fasting techniques. One person's solution might not be suitable for another. Be patient, continue to be open to trying new things, and give your body time to adjust to the new pattern.

We'll discuss how to incorporate intermittent fasting with a nutritious diet in the following chapter to enhance your general well-being and meet your health objectives.

Chapter 20: Combining Intermittent Fasting with a Healthful Diet

Congratulations on implementing intermittent fasting successfully into your way of life! Let's now look at how adding healthy, balanced food to your fasting regimen can increase its positive effects. Your intermittent fasting journey can be optimized and general well-being is promoted by proper nutrition. We'll explore the fundamentals of a wholesome diet that goes along with your fasting schedule in this chapter.

1. Emphasize Whole, Nutrient-Dense Foods

Prioritize whole, nutrient-dense foods that are high in antioxidants, vitamins, and minerals when you are breaking your fast. Include a lot of fresh produce in your meals, along with whole grains, lean proteins, and healthy fats. These foods support your body's nutritional needs as well as your energy levels and general health.

As much as possible, stay away from processed and sugary foods because they can cause sharp blood sugar increases and counteract the health benefits of fasting. If you must use artificial sweeteners, use natural ones like honey or maple syrup, but do so sparingly.

2. macronutrient balance

A balanced intake of the macronutrients carbs, proteins, and fats makes up a well-rounded diet. Energy is provided by carbohydrates, proteins help with muscle growth and repair, and healthy fats are necessary for several biological processes. To support your body's requirements, make sure that each meal has a balanced amount of these macronutrients.

4. Conscious Eating

Increasing one's level of food consciousness through intermittent fasting. When breaking your fast, take your time and enjoy every bite. Pay attention to your body's signals of hunger and fullness, and quit when you feel at ease. Eat sensibly throughout your eating window to avoid negating the advantages of fasting.

5. Planning and preparing meals

Planning and preparing your meals in advance can be quite beneficial when you are fasting. Prepare wholesome meals and snacks in advance to make sure you always have access to a variety of wholesome foods. This routine can help you stay on track with your fasting and nutritional objectives by preventing impulsive meal decisions.

6. dietary supplements

The majority of the nutrients your body needs should be covered by a well-balanced diet, but some people may benefit from taking certain nutritional supplements. To find out if you have any specific vitamin deficiencies or if supplements are required to support your general health, speak with a medical practitioner or registered dietitian.

7. Take Care of Yourself

Always keep in mind that progress, not perfection, is the goal of intermittent fasting. If you periodically stray from your fasting schedule or indulge in goodies, be compassionate to yourself and try not to feel needless guilt. The odd indulgence is acceptable and shouldn't detract from your dedication to living a healthy lifestyle in general.

8. Track Your Development

Keep track of your development as you mix intermittent fasting with a nutritious diet, as well as how your body adjusts to the changes. Keep a journal to record your mood, energy level, and any changes in your health or general well-being. You can determine what functions best for you using this practice, and you can also make any necessary adjustments.

9. Look for Community and Support

Finding a fasting companion or joining a community can inspire and encourage you on your quest. Together, share triumphs, trade advice, and celebrate experiences. The intermittent fasting experience can be more joyful and long-lasting if you have a support system.

You are providing your body with all the resources it needs to thrive by combining intermittent fasting with a wholesome diet. Improved energy, mental clarity, weight management, and general vigor can all be benefits of the synergistic interactions between fasting and healthy nutrition.

Chapter 21: Intermittent fasting for weight loss and fat burning

The ability of intermittent fasting to promote weight loss and fat burning is one of its most sought-after advantages. We'll explore the science of intermittent fasting in this chapter to see how it can support your weight reduction objectives and assist you in losing extra pounds.

1. Energy Deficiency

Fundamentally, weight loss happens when you eat fewer calories than your body uses. By reducing the amount of time you eat each day, intermittent fasting can help you naturally establish a calorie deficit. You may naturally consume fewer calories throughout the day by reducing your eating window, which will aid in weight loss.

Striking a balance is crucial to prevent severely limiting calories throughout your meal window. Emphasize nutrient-dense foods to give your body the vitamins and minerals it needs while still maintaining a calorie deficit.

2. Higher Fat Burning

Hormonal changes brought on by intermittent fasting improve the body's capacity to burn fat for energy. Insulin levels fall during fasting periods, facilitating the breakdown of body fat that has been accumulated. Your body may use stored fat for energy thanks to this metabolic change, which increases fat burning.

Furthermore, increased levels of the hormone norepinephrine, which is released when one fasts, promote the breakdown of fat cells. Accelerated fat loss is a result of elevated norepinephrine and decreased insulin.

3. **Lean muscle mass preservation**

Intermittent fasting has been demonstrated to help maintain lean muscle mass, in contrast, to crash diets that could cause muscle and fat loss simultaneously. Your body releases growth hormones when you limit your eating window; this hormone is essential for preserving and gaining muscle.

Regular resistance training and intermittent fasting can help maintain and build muscles even more. Exercises that increase your body's use of muscle tissue over fat as fuel result in a more toned and contoured figure.

4. **Appetite Control**

The effect of intermittent fasting on controlling appetite is one of its special advantages. According to some research, fasting may help lower levels of hunger hormones like ghrelin, which will lessen feelings of hunger. Keeping to your fasting schedule and avoiding overeating during your eating window may be made simpler as a result.

5. Permanent Weight Loss

Intermittent fasting differs from many conventional diets in that it can be maintained over time. Incorporating intermittent fasting into your lifestyle over time may be easier to handle and make it easier to maintain your weight reduction efforts.

6. Conscious Eating

A greater level of mindfulness when eating is fostered by intermittent fasting. You can have a healthier relationship with food by becoming more aware of your hunger and satiety cues. Your attempts to lose weight can be supported by mindful eating, which can help reduce emotional eating and impulsive food choices.

7. Individual Differences

It's important to understand that everyone experiences weight reduction differently. Your body's reaction to intermittent fasting can vary depending on your age, metabolism, amount of activity, and underlying medical issues. Keep trying and being patient, concentrating on your total health rather than just the figure on the scale.

8. In conjunction with exercise

While combining intermittent fasting with regular exercise can improve results, it can also help you lose weight. Strength training, aerobic activity, or a combination of the two can maximize fat-burning and advance general fitness.

Keep in mind that the purpose of intermittent fasting is to achieve permanent and healthy weight management, not merely immediate weight loss. It's a voyage that calls for endurance, reliability, and an emphasis on general health and well-being.

We'll examine how intermittent fasting can enhance your mental and emotional well-being in the following chapter, unlocking mental clarity and enhancing emotional well-being.

Chapter 22: The Mental and Emotional Advantages of Intermittent Fasting

Your mental and emotional health are significantly impacted by intermittent fasting, in addition to the physical aspects of your health. In this chapter, we'll examine how intermittent fasting might enhance your mental clarity, emotional stability, and overall well-being.

1. Improved Cognitive Function

According to studies, intermittent fasting can improve cognitive function and support brain health. Brain-derived neurotrophic factor (BDNF), a protein that promotes the growth and maintenance of nerve cells, is produced in greater quantities by the brain during fasting. Neuroplasticity, or the brain's capacity to change and create new connections, is vital for learning and memory.

Ketones, which are created during the breakdown of fats, may be produced in greater quantities during intermittent fasting. Ketones can act as a substitute energy source for the brain, offering a more reliable and effective fuel supply.

2. Mental Focus and Clarity

When engaging in intermittent fasting, many people claim to feel more focused and clear-headed. The inability to consume food continuously throughout the day may lessen blood sugar swings, stabilizing energy levels and mental alertness.

Additionally, since they are less preoccupied with thoughts and urges related to food when they are fasting, some people report that they are more productive. For tasks that demand sustained attention and concentration, this improved focus may be useful.

3. Regulation of Mood

The ability to control one's emotions and mood may also be affected by intermittent fasting. According to some research, fasting may help lower brain inflammation markers, which may lead to better mood and a lower risk of mood disorders.

Additionally, the endorphins that are released during fasting can produce feelings of joy and general well-being. Positive emotions are a result of many people reporting that they felt empowered and effective in sticking to their fasting routines.

4. Strength under Stress

Increased stress resilience has been linked to intermittent fasting. Fasting causes the activation of specific genes that support the body's ability to handle stress and defend against its damaging consequences. An increase in emotional stability and better stress management may result from this adaptive reaction.

5. Aware of Emotional Eating

People who intermittently fast may become more conscious of their emotional eating habits. People can create healthy coping methods and lessen emotional eating by paying attention to and understanding the relationship between emotions and eating behaviors.

Individuals who learn to enjoy their meals and concentrate on fueling their bodies might benefit from mindful eating practices throughout the eating window, which can enhance emotional well-being.

6. sleeping well

Some people discover that intermittent fasting improves the quality of their sleep. More peaceful and rejuvenating sleep may be encouraged by stable blood sugar levels during fasting periods and a potential rise in melatonin production.

7. Developing Resilience

It takes discipline and persistence to perform intermittent fasting. A sense of resilience and self-control that goes beyond dietary preferences and positively impacts other facets of life can be fostered by adopting this lifestyle adjustment.

Although many people find that intermittent fasting improves their mental and emotional health, individual reactions can differ. It's critical to proceed with caution and get advice from a healthcare provider if you have a history of disordered eating or other mental health issues.

The benefits of intermittent fasting for many elements of physical health, such as hormone control and metabolism, will be discussed in more detail in the following chapter.

Chapter 23: Intermittent Fasting to Increase Muscle and Strength

When used in conjunction with the appropriate techniques, intermittent fasting can assist in strength and muscular improvements in addition to weight loss. We'll look at how intermittent fasting can be modified to encourage muscle growth and enhance your fitness journey in this chapter.

1. Timing and Intake of Protein

The timing and amount of protein consumed are key for maximizing the potential for muscle growth and repair. Concentrate on eating enough foods high in protein during your eating window. To provide a consistent supply of amino acids to your muscles, aim for a balanced distribution of protein throughout your meals.

According to research, ingesting protein soon after working out can be especially advantageous for muscle growth and rehabilitation. To take advantage of the window for muscle growth, think about eating a protein-rich meal or snack soon after your workout.

2. Resistance Exercise

To promote muscular growth, resistance training, such as weightlifting or bodyweight exercises, is crucial. By maximizing the hormonal responses that drive muscle growth, intermittent fasting can enhance your resistance training program.

Human growth hormone (HGH) levels frequently rise during fasting intervals, which may improve muscle protein synthesis. Greater muscular gains may result from combining resistance training with this natural HGH increase.

3. Vitamin Timing

When using intermittent fasting, careful nutrition scheduling can further boost muscle building. Consider scheduling your workouts for the last few hours of your fast, right before you break it. In this manner, you can maximize your muscles' post-workout recuperation by giving them nutrients right away.

4. Caloric Overage During Mealtime

While calorie deficits produced by intermittent fasting can aid in weight loss, people who want to gain muscle may need to ingest more calories during their meal window. Consuming more calories than your body needs to produce the energy and building blocks for muscular growth is known as a caloric surplus.

Remember that a caloric surplus should come from foods that are high in nutrients rather than from empty calories. To encourage the growth of muscles and overall health, emphasize wholesome sources of proteins, lipids, and carbs.

6. Ample Rest and Recuperation

Additionally, enough rest and recovery are necessary for muscular growth. Make sure you receive adequate sleep every night to aid in the body's natural recovery and muscle regeneration processes. Additionally, taking rest days in between strenuous workouts might help avoid overtraining and improve outcomes.

7. Consistency and Patience

Muscle-building is a gradual process that calls for consistency and patience. Over time, it's crucial to stick to your resistance training regimen and keep up a regular fasting schedule. Keep track of your development and reward minor victories along the road to maintain motivation.

8. Avoid Very Tight Calorie Limits

While significant calorie limitations during the eating window should be avoided, intermittent fasting can be compatible with muscle growth. Calorie restriction to an extreme might impede muscle growth and recovery, producing less-than-ideal results.

Keep in mind that each person's body is different and that different people may react differently to intermittent fasting. It's crucial to pay attention to your body and change your strategy as necessary to support your unique fitness goals.

We'll examine how intermittent fasting can help longevity, anti-aging, and general health in the following chapter.

Chapter 24: Intermittent fasting and metabolic health

Intermittent fasting can have a significant impact on metabolic health, which is vital for general health and plays a role in intermittent fasting. We'll look at how intermittent fasting affects many areas of metabolism and energy management in this chapter.

1. Power Balance

By encouraging a caloric deficit during fasting periods, intermittent fasting aids in the regulation of energy balance. One can assist in weight loss and maintain a healthier energy balance by ingesting fewer calories during a constrained eating window.

2. Insulin Control

One important hormone that controls blood sugar levels is insulin. A reduction in the risk of insulin resistance and type 2 diabetes can be achieved with intermittent fasting, which increases insulin sensitivity.

3. Blood Sugar Metabolism

The body uses glucose that has been stored as fuel when fasting. This procedure can enhance glucose metabolism and aid in blood sugar level stabilization.

4. Fat Loss with Ketosis

The metabolic state of ketosis, in which the body utilizes stored fat as its main source of energy, can be brought on by intermittent fasting. Weight loss is supported by ketosis, which also promotes fat burning.

5. Profile of Lipids

By lowering levels of LDL cholesterol (the "bad" cholesterol) and triglycerides while raising levels of HDL cholesterol (the "good" cholesterol), intermittent fasting may enhance lipid profiles.

6. Metabolic Adjustment

The ability of the body to switch between using various fuel sources, such as glucose and lipids, for energy, is referred to as metabolic flexibility. By teaching the body to switch between various energy sources quickly and effectively, intermittent fasting encourages metabolic flexibility.

7. Metabolic Rate at Rest

According to several studies, intermittent fasting may not have a substantial effect on resting metabolic rate or the number of calories burnt while at rest. As it maintains energy expenditure during fasting periods, this may be advantageous.

8. Body's microbiome

The community of bacteria that live in the digestive system, known as the gut microbiome, can be affected by intermittent fasting. The efficient functioning of digestion and metabolism depends on a healthy gut microbiota.

9. Mitochondrial Activity

The organelles in cells that produce energy are called mito-chondria. By boosting mitochondrial efficiency and function, intermittent fasting may improve overall energy control.

10. Permanent Metabolic Advantages

Intermittent fasting has benefits for metabolism that go beyond the fasting windows. Intermittent fasting may improve overall metabolic health and result in long-term metabolic improve-ments.

While intermittent fasting can have a variety of positive effects on metabolic health, individual responses may differ. Age, genetics, and general health state are just a few examples of variables that may affect how intermittent fasting affects metabolism.

The practical components of intermittent fasting, including how to get started, typical difficulties, and how to maintain intermittent fasting as a long-term habit, will be covered in the following chapter.

Chapter 25: Intermittent Fasting: A Practical Guide

Now that you are aware of the numerous advantages of intermittent fasting, it is time to investigate how you may practically adopt this way of living into your everyday routine. We'll give you a step-by-step manual in this chapter to assist you begin intermittent fasting and get past frequent obstacles.

1. Select the Proper Intermittent Fasting Technique

There are several widely used forms of intermittent fasting, each with a different strategy for fasting and eating windows. Typical techniques include:

- The 16/8 Method is a daily 8-hour interval for eating followed by a 16-hour fast.

- 5:2 Approach: Consume regularly five days per week while drastically reducing calorie intake (by 500–600 calories) on two separate days.

- Stop-Eat-Eat: Once or twice per week, fast for a full 24 hours.

- Alternate-Day Fasting: Alternate between days when you

fast and days when you normally eat.

- Warrior Diet: Eat one huge meal at night and fast during the day.

Pick a strategy that fits your preferences and way of life. It's sometimes advised to start with the 16/8 approach if you're new to intermittent fasting because it's reasonably simple to use.

2. Gradual Change

If you're new to intermittent fasting, think about easing into longer fasts instead of doing so all at once. Start by progressively lengthening the interval between dinner and morning. This strategy enables your body to adjust to the fasting schedule more easily.

3. Maintain hydration

Maintaining hydration is crucial when fasting. Drink lots of water, herbal teas, and unsweetened black coffee to stay healthy. Proper hydration can assist your body's natural detoxification processes and help you feel fuller longer.

4. Create A Balanced Diet

Prioritize balanced meals that offer the required nutrients when breaking your fast. A variety of whole foods, such as fruits, vegetables, lean meats, and healthy fats, should be consumed. When eating, try to limit your intake of processed and sugary meals.

5. Pay Attention to Your Body

Pay heed to your body's signals of hunger and fullness. It's about developing a healthy and sustainable eating routine; intermittent fasting is not about deprivation or intense hunger. You should modify your fasting schedule if you feel sick or overly hungry.

6. Preparing meals

During intermittent fasting, it can be quite helpful to plan and prepare meals in advance. Having healthy options close at hand might help you avoid compulsive eating decisions and make keeping to your fasting schedule easier.

7. Physical exercise and activity

Make regular exercise a part of your regimen. Although you can work out when you're fasting, some people arrange their workouts during their eating windows for the best performance and recuperation.

8. Overcoming Difficulties

There may be difficulties with intermittent fasting, especially at first. Hunger pangs, social settings involving food, and changing bad eating habits are all frequent obstacles. Keep in mind that you may experience some challenges at first, but they frequently grow easier to handle as you become used to the fasting routine.

10. **Sustainability Over Time**

Instead of treating intermittent fasting like a temporary diet, consider it a lifestyle change. For intermittent fasting to be effective, it must be sustained and practiced regularly.

Chapter 26: Success Stories of Intermittent Fasting

Worldwide, intermittent fasting has become more and more popular, and countless people have adopted it with impressive results. In this chapter, we'll present uplifting success tales from real people who have used intermittent fasting to noticeably enhance their health and general well-being.

Sarah's Weight Loss Experience 1

Years of unsuccessful diet attempts by Sarah contributed to her inability to regulate her weight. She learned about intermittent fasting and decided to try it. Beginning with the 16/8 technique, Sarah progressively changed her eating window and meal preferences.

Sarah observed a significant reduction in her weight and the number of inches around her waist within a few months. But more importantly, she felt more energized and sharper mentally. Her connection with food was revolutionized by intermittent fasting, which also assisted her in losing extra weight and helped her adopt a more conscious and balanced eating style.

2. John's Transformation in Fitness

John, a fitness enthusiast, was looking for strategies to improve his efficiency and muscle development. He made intermittent fasting a part of his habit, eating later in the day after breaking his fast in the morning and early afternoon.

John was surprised to discover that intermittent fasting not only helped him achieve his muscle-building objectives but also increased his general energy and training endurance. He developed a more toned body composition, and he recovered more quickly after challenging workouts. Today, John considers intermittent fasting to be a crucial part of his fitness path.

3. Emily's Better Digestive Health

Emily frequently experienced bloating and discomfort after meals as a result of digestive problems. She decided to give intermittent fasting a go as a possible remedy. Emily discovered that her gut health significantly improved when she gave her digestive system longer intervals in between meals.

Emily reported decreased bloating and gastrointestinal discomfort when she practiced intermittent fasting. She learned that her body thrived with a longer nighttime fast, and her digestion improved and became more regular.

Tom's Improved Mental Acuity

Tom was a busy worker who frequently experienced mental tiredness and drowsiness throughout long workdays. His mental clarity and attentiveness much improved after he started intermittent fasting.

Tom had consistent energy levels throughout the day by avoiding frequent snacking and keeping his eating window narrowed to nutrient-dense foods. He was able to remain focused and productive during his busy workday via intermittent fasting.

5. Mary's Balanced Hormones

Mary had experienced mood swings and irregular cycles as a result of hormone imbalances. She decided to experiment with intermittent fasting to support hormone balance under the advice of her healthcare professional.

She was pleased to find that the hormonal balance had improved with intermittent fasting. Her menstrual cycle became more regular, and her mood swings diminished. Mary's strategy for promoting the health and well-being of her hormones was enhanced by intermittent fasting.

6. James' Better Blood Sugar Management

James, who has type 2 diabetes, was looking for better ways to control his blood sugar levels. Under the guidance of his medical staff, he started intermittent fasting and experienced notable improvements.

James was able to lessen his reliance on diabetic medication and maintain his blood sugar levels with intermittent fasting and a healthy diet. His diabetes treatment strategy began to benefit greatly from intermittent fasting.

7. Lily's Feeling of Power

Lily had a difficult relationship with food and suffered from emotional eating. She was able to free herself from emotional eating behaviors and restore control over her eating habits thanks to intermittent fasting.

Lily developed a more conscious eating style after discovering how to distinguish between emotional and physical hunger through intermittent fasting. Her ability to follow a fasting schedule and make healthy decisions while eating was empowering to her.

These are just a few instances of how intermittent fasting has a positive impact on people's lives. It's important to understand that everyone's experience with intermittent fasting is different. Consult a healthcare provider before beginning intermittent fasting, especially if you have any underlying medical ailments or worries.

Chapter 27: Intermittent Fasting A Healthy Lifestyle

L et's review the most important lessons learned from the experience of intermittent fasting and how it can improve your health and well-being as we wrap up this book.

1. A Flexible Strategy

A flexible and adaptive approach to nutrition and health is provided by intermittent fasting. People can discover a fasting plan that fits their lifestyle and tastes by selecting from a variety of fasting techniques.

2. Dietary Control and Fat Loss

The management of weight and the reduction of fat may be accomplished by intermittent fasting. Intermittent fasting helps people lose weight in a healthy and long-lasting way by encouraging metabolic changes and a calorie deficit.

3. Gains in strength and muscle mass

Intermittent fasting and resistance training can help people who want to increase their strength and improve their sports performance to expand their muscles.

4. Cognitive ability and brain health

Positive effects of intermittent fasting on brain health include improved memory, mental acuity, and cognitive performance. The enhancement of neuroplasticity and an increase in BDNF both help the brain function better.

5. Longevity and Heart Health

Various heart health advantages of intermittent fasting have been linked to it, including better lipid profiles, blood pressure, and lower inflammation. Its putative anti-aging benefits could increase longevity in general.

6. Metabolic Health

Intermittent fasting promotes overall metabolic health and blood sugar control by altering lipid profiles, glucose metabolism, and insulin sensitivity.

7. Emotional intelligence and mindful eating

Intermittent fasting can promote attentive eating habits and help people learn to recognize their hunger and satiety cues. It might also make people more conscious of their emotional eating habits.

8. Considerations for Individualization and Health

Depending on factors like age, genetics, and general health status, each person's response to intermittent fasting may differ. Before beginning intermittent fasting, it's critical to take into account your individual needs and seek advice from a healthcare provider.

9. Sustainable Way of Life

Instead of being on a quick-fix diet, intermittent fasting is a healthy way of life. People can find long-lasting advantages for their health and well-being by making intermittent fasting a long-term commitment.

10. Individual Power

Intermittent fasting, according to many people, gives them the power to take charge of their health and create lasting changes in their life. People can gain a better awareness of their bodies and relationships with food by adopting this lifestyle.

Keep in mind that doing an intermittent fast is just one method of achieving a healthy lifestyle. Intermittent fasting can be used as part of a comprehensive and holistic approach to health when combined with regular exercise, a healthy diet, and self-care routines.

Be kind to yourself as you start your intermittent fasting adventure and recognize your accomplishments along the way. Your dedication to achieving the highest level of health and well-being is demonstrated by each step you take.

We appreciate your participation in our exploration of inter-mittent fasting. I wish you happiness, empowerment, and fulfillment on your journey to health.

III

The Ultimate Guide to the Keto Diet: Achieving Health and Weight Loss

"Embrace the power of the keto diet – fueling your body with determination and ketones, one transformative choice at a time."

Introduction

P lease accept my sincere welcome to "The Ultimate Guide to the Keto Diet: Achieving Health and Weight Loss"! This extensive book will cover all the information you require regarding the ketogenic diet, a high-fat, low-carb eating regimen that has become incredibly popular in recent years.

We will explore the various facets of the keto diet chapter by chapter, giving you a solid foundation of information to support your weight reduction and health objectives. This book is intended to be a helpful resource that covers all the necessary knowledge, useful advice, and delectable recipes to make your keto journey a success, whether you're a novice or have some experience with keto.

Chapter 28: Understanding the Ketogenic Diet

The low-carb, high-fat ketogenic diet, sometimes known as the keto diet, has grown significantly in popularity in recent years. It is intended to change your body's metabolism such that fat is used as your body's primary fuel source instead of carbs as its primary energy source. The keto diet tries to bring about a state of ketosis by substantially reducing your carbohydrate intake and boosting your intake of healthy fats.

When glucose (produced from carbohydrates) is scarce, your body naturally creates ketones from fat stores to supply energy. This process is known as ketosis. Your body becomes very effective at using stored body fat as fuel while you are in ketosis, which causes weight loss and improves your body's composition.

The ketogenic diet's main macronutrient ratios are typically 70–75% calories from fat, 20–25% calories from protein, and 10–20% calories from carbohydrates. Individual needs may vary, but by severely limiting carbohydrates to less than 50 grams per day, the body exhausts its glycogen reserves and enters ketosis within a few days to a week.

The keto diet places a strong emphasis on eating healthy fats, which is one of the primary characteristics that set it apart from other low-carb eating plans. Avocados, nuts, seeds, and fatty fish are a few examples of foods high in monounsaturated and polyunsaturated fats that should be consumed. The keto diet also accepts saturated fats, such as those found in coconut oil, grass-fed butter, and full-fat dairy products. Trans fats and heavily processed vegetable oils ought to be avoided, nevertheless.

For the ketogenic diet to be successfully implemented, it is essential to comprehend the science underlying it. Your body's insulin levels fall when you limit carbohydrates, which reduces fat accumulation and increases fat breakdown. To give other organs, including the brain, a consistent source of energy, the liver starts to make ketones from fatty acids.

The ketogenic diet has several possible health advantages besides weight loss. It is advantageous for people with type 2 diabetes or those who are at risk of getting it because it has shown promise in improving insulin sensitivity and blood sugar control. The diet may also improve mental clarity and concentration since ketones can give the brain a more reliable and effective energy source. According to certain research, the ketogenic diet may have anti-inflammatory properties that lower the chance of developing chronic diseases.

It's vital to remember that not everyone should follow a ketogenic diet. People with specific illnesses, like pancreatitis or liver disease, should avoid the diet or speak with their doctor before beginning. The keto diet should also be used with caution by individuals who are expecting or nursing, as well as by those who have a history of disordered eating.

In summary, the ketogenic diet encourages ketosis, a metabolic state in which the body burns fat for fuel. It is a low-carb, high-fat diet. People may decide whether the keto diet is a good fit for their health and weight reduction objectives by knowing the fundamental ideas underlying the diet and how it affects metabolism. A healthcare practitioner should be consulted before making any dietary changes to provide individualized advice and assistance.

Chapter 29: Ketosis's Scientific Basis

We will go more into the science of ketosis, the metabolic state that the ketogenic diet seeks to produce, in this chapter. Understanding how the body switches from using glucose as its primary fuel source to depending on ketones obtained from fat is crucial for understanding the mechanisms involved in ketosis.

When you eat a conventional diet that contains carbohydrates, your body converts those carbohydrates into glucose as part of the digestive process. The blood then carries the glucose to the cells, where it is used as an energy source. The pancreas' hormone insulin aids in controlling blood glucose levels.

However, the body's ability to access glucose is constrained when carbohydrate consumption is markedly reduced, as is the situation with the ketogenic diet. The body must therefore locate a different source of energy to maintain its operations. Ketosis has a role in this situation.

When the liver starts converting fatty acids into ketone bodies, ketosis sets in. Beta-hydroxybutyrate (BHB), acetoacetate, and acetone are three types of ketone bodies that can be carried in the bloodstream to supply energy to different bodily tissues, including the brain.

When fatty acids from stored fat are converted into fatty acids through a process known as lipolysis, the synthesis of ketone bodies begins. The liver continues to break down these fatty acids, resulting in the creation of ketone bodies. When dietary carbohydrate consumption is low and dietary fat availability is high, the liver can produce ketones more quickly.

Once they are created, ketones act as the body's alternate fuel source. Ketones, as opposed to glucose, can effectively pass the blood-brain barrier, giving the brain a quick source of energy. This is one reason why people who are in a state of ketosis frequently report having more mental clarity and attention.

Additionally, a variety of tissues use ketones as an energy source, including heart and muscle cells. This enables the body to save glucose for tissues that depend on it, like red blood cells and specific regions of the brain that are unable to use ketones properly.

The body experiences several physiological changes when it enters ketosis and switches to ketone metabolism. First off, once carbohydrate intake is decreased, insulin levels fall. This encourages fat breakdown and prevents fat storage. This is why the ketogenic diet is frequently successful in reducing body fat and promoting weight loss.

Blood sugar levels are also impacted by ketosis. The body needs less glucose while it is in a ketosis condition, which lessens the requirement for significant insulin releases after meals. For those who have diabetes or insulin resistance, this may be advantageous as it can aid with blood sugar regulation.

The body's hormone levels are impacted by ketosis. To maintain glucose homeostasis, insulin, and glucagon, another hormone involved in controlling blood sugar levels, cooperate. During ketosis, there is a decrease in insulin levels, which causes a rise in glucagon release. The breakdown of liver glycogen (glucose storage) and subsequent synthesis of ketones are both influenced by the interaction of hormones.

The ketogenic diet has also been shown to have anti-inflammatory properties. Numerous illnesses, such as heart disease, diabetes, and neurological disorders, are linked to chronic inflammation. The diet may help modify inflammatory pathways in the body, perhaps providing protective effects, by lowering carbohydrate intake and encouraging ketosis.

While many people can benefit from ketosis, it may not be appropriate for everyone, it is crucial to keep in mind. Before attempting a ketogenic diet, some medical issues, such as pancreatitis or liver illness, may need careful attention. To ascertain whether the diet is suitable for you and to guarantee thorough monitoring of any underlying health issues, you must consult with a healthcare practitioner.

In conclusion, the metabolic state of ketosis occurs when the body switches from using glucose as its primary fuel source to utilizing ketones obtained from fat. People may grasp the mechanisms by which the ketogenic diet causes this state and the potential advantages it offers for weight reduction, blood sugar control, and inflammatory modulation by studying the science of ketosis. To make sure the diet fits specific needs and goals, it is crucial to get individualized advice and support from healthcare specialists as with any dietary adjustment.

Chapter 30: Benefits of the Keto Diet

This chapter will examine the several advantages of the ketogenic diet that go beyond weight loss. While many people's main objective with the keto diet is to reach and maintain a healthy weight, it also has several other benefits that improve general well-being.

1. Weight Loss: The keto diet is well known for helping people lose weight. The body enters a state of ketosis, where it uses stored fat as its main fuel source, by dramatically reducing carbohydrate intake and boosting healthy fat consumption. As a result, there may be a decrease in body fat, an improvement in body composition, and effective long-term weight management.

2. Increased Mental Clarity and Focus: The brain consumes a lot of energy. Ketones act as a more reliable and effective source of energy for the brain than glucose when the body is in a state of ketosis. Many people who follow the ketogenic diet claim to have a better cognitive function, mental clarity, and attention, which can be especially helpful for tasks that call for concentration and mental acuity.

3. Increased Energy Levels: The body uses stored body fat and dietary fat more effectively when it switches from using carbohydrates to fat as fuel. Avoiding the energy dumps sometimes brought on by changes in blood sugar levels that occur with high-carbohydrate diets, can lead to maintaining energy levels throughout the day.

4. Reduced Hunger and Cravings: The high-fat, moderate-protein foods that are emphasized by the keto diet tend to encourage fullness and lessen sensations of hunger. Generally speaking, healthy fats and proteins are more gratifying and filling than carbohydrates, which reduces the desire for frequent snacking and overeating. This may make it simpler to follow a diet plan and maintain calorie restriction.

5. Improved Blood Sugar Control: Eating carbohydrates affects blood sugar levels directly, with high-carb meals causing glucose rises and insulin releases. The low-carb characteristic of the keto diet can aid in blood sugar stabilization and increase insulin sensitivity. For people with type 2 diabetes or those who are at risk of getting the disease, this is very advantageous.

6. Potential Therapeutic Uses: The ketogenic diet has demonstrated potential in several therapeutic uses beyond weight loss. Epilepsy, particularly in kids with drug-resistant seizures, metabolic syndrome, and polycystic ovarian syndrome (PCOS), according to research, may all benefit from it. Before using the diet as a therapeutic intervention, it is crucial to get the advice of medical experts.

7. Effects on Inflammation: Chronic inflammation is linked to

several diseases, including diabetes, heart disease, and several autoimmune disorders. It has been discovered that the keto-genic diet has anti-inflammatory properties, possibly lowering inflammatory markers in the body. The diet may lead to an improvement in general health by minimizing the consumption of pro-inflammatory processed foods and encouraging the intake of anti-inflammatory fats and nutrients.

8. Potential Benefits for Brain Health: It has been demonstrated that the production of ketones during ketosis gives the brain a different energy source. This has sparked curiosity in the keto diet's possible application to treat neurological diseases includ-ing Parkinson's and Alzheimer's. Although additional research is required in this area, preliminary studies suggest potential advantages for mental health and cognitive performance.

9. Improvements in Physical Performance: Although the body predominantly requires carbohydrates for high-intensity ac-tivity, several athletes and endurance enthusiasts have claimed better performance after adjusting to a keto diet. The body's capacity to use fat as a source of energy effectively can be help-ful in some circumstances, such as long-duration endurance sports.

10. Long-Term Health and Wellness: The keto diet promotes the consumption of nutrient-dense foods like veggies, healthy fats, and lean meats by lowering dependency on processed carbohydrates and sweets. This may result in enhanced general dietary habits and long-term health and well-being.

It is significant to remember that each person may react differently to the keto diet, and not everyone will enjoy all of its advantages. Additionally, those who are pregnant or nursing as well as those with specific medical issues may not be able to follow the ketogenic diet. Before beginning any significant dietary changes, it is imperative to seek the counsel of medical professionals and receive specialized guidance.

In conclusion, the ketogenic diet has several advantages outside of weight loss, such as improved mental clarity, more energy, better blood sugar regulation, and possible therapeutic uses. Its attractiveness is also boosted by its anti-inflammatory properties, possible advantages for brain health, and beneficial impacts on athletic performance. However, it is crucial to take into account unique situations, speak with healthcare professionals, and make decisions that are based on individual health objectives and needs.

Chapter 31: Setting Your Goals

When starting the ketogenic diet or any other nutritional modification, setting definite, attainable goals is crucial. You can maintain focus, drive, and a clear sense of progress by setting your goals in advance. We will examine the essential elements of goal planning in this chapter to assist you in beginning your keto journey.

1. Define Your Goals: Explain why you want to follow the ketogenic diet in the beginning. Are weight loss, increased energy, better blood sugar regulation, or general health and wellness your top priorities? Understanding your goals will enable you to adjust your strategy and adhere to your objectives throughout the process.

2. Be explicit and Measurable: To properly track your progress, set explicit goals that can be measured. Instead of saying, "I want to lose weight," for instance, be more specific about how much weight you want to drop and when you want to do it. This gives you a specific goal to work toward and enables you to monitor your development as you go.

3. Set Reasonable Expectations: Although the ketogenic diet has

many advantages, it's crucial to have reasonable expectations. For instance, rapid and long-lasting weight loss usually occurs at a rate of 1-2 pounds each week. Prioritizing long-term, sustainable reforms over a narrow focus on immediate results is crucial.

4. Break It Down: Separate your objectives into more manageable, attainable milestones. Your goals will be less intimidating if you break them down into doable milestones, and you'll feel more accomplished as you reach each one. Celebrating these modest successes can keep motivation and momentum going.

5. Make a timetable: Create a timetable for your objectives and assign due dates to each milestone. This gives the situation a sense of urgency and offers a system for monitoring development. Though every person's path is different, it's crucial to prioritize consistency and durability over strict time limits, so be flexible with your timeframe.

6. Though weight loss is frequently a top priority, keep in mind to recognize and celebrate non-scale successes as well. Progress is best measured by rising energy levels, bettering sleep quality, increasing mental acuity, and raising physical performance. Pay attention to these successes and acknowledge them as you go.

7. Personalize Your Goals: Adapt your goals to your unique requirements and situation. When selecting your goals, take into account things like your lifestyle, tastes, and present state of health. Make sure your goals are reasonable and appropriate for your particular scenario because what works for someone else might not work for you.

8. Seek Support: Discuss your objectives with dependable family members, close friends, or a support group. Having a support network can offer inspiration, responsibility, and insightful advice. Finding a keto buddy or joining an online community can both provide support and assistance for your journey.

9. Keep a diary of your progress to track your accomplishments and pinpoint areas that require improvement. This can be achieved in several ways, such as by keeping a journal or by keeping track of your food intake, physical activity, and energy levels. By regularly assessing your progress, you may make the required corrections and maintain your motivation.

10. Maintain Flexibility and Adaptability: As you advance along your keto journey, keep in mind that goals may change over time. Pay attention to your body, be willing to make modifications, and enjoy the process of learning. Your objectives may change in response to fresh information, evolving circumstances, or individual preferences. The secret is to keep an open mind and carry on making decisions that are in line with your health and happiness.

In conclusion, success with the ketogenic diet depends on defining specific, attainable goals. You may maintain motivation and attention by setting your goals, dividing them into smaller milestones, and monitoring your progress. Along the journey, don't forget to celebrate both scale- and non-scale wins, personalize your goals, and look for support. Accept flexibility and adaptability

The Ultimate 28-Day Keto Meal Plan: Transform Your Health and Body

Are you ready to take a leap towards a healthier and slimmer body? This 28-day Keto Meal Plan is the perfect guide to help you reach your health and fitness goals. This comprehensive plan is designed to help you transition into the ketogenic lifestyle, which is a low-carb, high-fat diet that puts your body into a state of ketosis. During this process, your body will switch from relying on glucose for energy to burning stored fats, leading to effective weight loss and a range of health benefits.

Week 1: Day 1
  Breakfast: eggs with avocado and spinach scrambled.
  Lunch will be a grilled chicken salad with cucumbers, mixed greens, and an olive oil dressing.
  Dinner will be baked fish with mashed cauliflower and asparagus.

Day 2:
  Greek yogurt for breakfast with berries and chopped almonds
  Lunch would be lettuce wraps with tuna salad, mayo, and celery.
  Dinner will be beef stir-fry with bell peppers, broccoli, and sesame oil.

Day 3:
  Eggs and bacon for breakfast.
  Lunch consists of grilled shrimp over zucchini noodles with pesto sauce.

Grilled steak, roasted Brussels sprouts, and a side salad for dinner.

Day 4:

Chia seed pudding for breakfast with coconut milk and vanilla essence

Egg salad for lunch with mayo, mustard, and dill

Dinner will be garlic-butter baked chicken thighs with green beans.

Day 5:

Breakfast smoothie made with spinach, almond butter, protein powder, and almond milk.

Lunch will be lettuce wraps with avocado, bacon, tomato, and ranch dressing.

Dinner will consist of pork chops, roasted cauliflower, and sautéed spinach.

Day 6:

Breakfast: a cheese, mushroom, and bell pepper omelet

Lunch consists of a handmade Caesar salad with chicken.

Dinner will consist of grilled fish, broccoli, and cauliflower rice.

Day 7:

Cottage cheese with sliced strawberries and walnuts for breakfast

Lunch: lettuce wraps with turkey, avocado, mayo, and mustard

Baked eggplant for dinner Salad on the side and parmesan.

Week 2: Fueling Your Keto Fire

Maintain a rotation of varied protein and vegetable choices, incorporating various tastes and textures. Do not forget to consume healthy fats such as avocado, olive oil, and almonds. Be aware of your daily carbohydrate intake and aim for 20 to 50 grams.

Day 14: Power-Packed Lunch

Make lunchtime a culinary adventure with a keto-friendly Cobb salad. Crisp lettuce, succulent grilled chicken, crispy bacon, and a drizzle of tangy ranch dressing create a symphony of flavors and textures that will keep you satisfied and energized.

Week 3: Mastering the Art of Keto Cooking

Day 21: Exquisite Dinner Delight

Dinner takes on a gourmet twist with a perfectly seared steak adorned with garlic butter. Paired with a side of sautéed asparagus and cauliflower mash, this meal showcases the elegance of keto dining while ensuring you stay on track.

Week 4: Achieving Keto Excellence

Day 28: Culmination Celebration

As you approach the end of your 28-day keto journey, it's time to celebrate your achievements. Whip up a batch of fluffy keto pancakes for breakfast, topped with a dollop of sugar-free whipped cream and a sprinkle of dark chocolate shavings.

In conclusion, our 28-day Keto Meal Plan is your key to a healthier, more vibrant you. With carefully crafted meals and a focus on nutrient-dense, delicious foods, you'll experience the incredible benefits of the ketogenic lifestyle. Say goodbye to excess weight and hello to renewed vitality – your journey to optimal health starts now. Remember, each meal is a step closer to your goals, and with dedication and our comprehensive plan, success is within reach. Are you ready to transform your life through the power of keto? The choice is yours.

Chapter 32: Keto-Friendly Foods & Meal Planning

A ketogenic diet entails reorienting your eating habits to put high-fat, low-carb foods first. We will examine a variety of keto-friendly foods in this chapter and offer advice on meal preparation to help you keep a healthy, fulfilling diet while remaining in ketosis.

Suitable Meals for Keto:

1. Healthy Fats: A successful ketogenic diet depends on a focus on healthy fats. Include items like avocados, olive, coconut, nuts and seeds, grass-fed butter, salmon, and other fatty seafood. These fats help several body processes, give energy, and encourage satiety.

2. Select high-quality sources of protein such as eggs, poultry, lean meats, fish, and seafood. For the upkeep and healing of muscles, protein is crucial. Aim for a reasonable protein intake because too much protein can prevent ketosis.

3. Low-Carb Vegetables: Non-starchy vegetables are a great option for a keto diet because they are high in fiber and low

in carbohydrates. Leafy greens (spinach, kale, lettuce), bell peppers, broccoli, cauliflower, zucchini, and asparagus are other examples. These vegetables contribute to the nutritional variety and offer vital nutrients.

4. Full-Fat Dairy: Choose full-fat dairy items instead of their low-fat counterparts. Examples include cheese, yogurt, and heavy cream (in moderation). Be aware of how your body reacts to dairy, though, as some people may need to restrict or avoid it owing to lactose intolerance or other allergies.

5. Nuts and seeds are nutrient-dense foods that offer fiber, healthy fats, and minerals as snacks. You should include foods like almonds, walnuts, chia seeds, flaxseeds, and hemp seeds in your diet. Because they are high in calories, pay attention to portion amounts.

6. Fruits are normally higher in carbohydrates than berries, but because of their reduced sugar content, berries like strawberries, raspberries, and blackberries can be consumed in moderation on a ketogenic diet. Take advantage of them as a sweet treat or as a yogurt topping in moderation.

7. Spices and herbs: Because they are essentially carb-free, spices and herbs can enhance the flavor of your food. Spices like basil, oregano, rosemary, cinnamon, and turmeric give your meals variety and depth without interfering with ketosis.

Meal preparation:

1. Determine Your Macronutrient Ratios: Based on your unique

needs and goals, calculate your macronutrient ratios. The keto diet often calls for ingesting 70–75% of calories as fat, 20–25% as protein, and 10–15% as carbohydrates. To fit your particular needs, alter these percentages as necessary.

2. Create your meal plans around keto-friendly ingredients. Include non-starchy veggies, a source of protein (meat, fish, or eggs), and healthy fats (oils, butter, avocado). To ensure a varied intake of nutrients, strive for a variety of hues and flavors.

3. Keep Track of Your Carbohydrate Intake: To stay within the ideal range, keep track of your daily carbohydrate intake. Be aware of hidden carbohydrates in processed meals, sauces, and condiments. When possible, choose entire, unprocessed meals.

4. While the keto diet restricts carbohydrates, fiber-rich foods like non-starchy vegetables, nuts, and seeds should be given priority. Fiber enhances general gut health, facilitates digestion, and increases satiety.

5. Meal preparation: To save time and make sure you have keto-friendly options available, think about meal preparation. To make quick meals throughout the week, prepare large portions of proteins, vegetables, and healthy fats in advance.

6. Make wise snacking decisions to control hunger and prevent reaching for high-carb foods between meals. Nuts, seeds, cheese, hard-boiled eggs, and small servings of low-carb vegetables with dip are among the options.

7. Keep Hydrated: On a ketogenic diet, being properly hydrated

is crucial. to assist digestion, control body temperature, and maintain general health, drink lots of water throughout the day.

8. Look for recipe inspiration by browsing cookbooks, internet resources, and websites with keto-friendly recipes. To make your meals pleasurable and avoid boredom, experiment with various tastes and cooking methods.

Always pay attention to your body's signals and modify your meal selections and portion sizes to your unique requirements and objectives. Consult with qualified dietitians or medical specialists frequently to make sure you're getting the nutrition you need while on the ketogenic diet.

In conclusion, an effective ketogenic diet incorporates low-carb veggies, moderate protein, and foods high in healthy fats. You may prepare filling and varied meals while keeping your body in a state of ketosis by practicing thoughtful meal planning, portion management, and an emphasis on nutrient-dense foods.

Chapter 33: Shopping for Success in the Grocery Store

Making the appropriate decisions at the grocery store is the first step to successfully implementing a ketogenic diet. We will give you useful advice and techniques in this chapter so that you can shop wisely, choose keto-friendly foods, and position yourself for success.

1. Make a detailed shopping list based on your meal plan and the foods that are keto-friendly before you go to the store. You can stay focused and prevent impulsive buying of non-keto items by doing this.

2. Shop the Perimeter: Fresh, whole foods are often found outside of supermarkets. Produce, meat and seafood counters, and dairy goods are all included in this. While the center aisles tend to include more processed and carb-heavy goods, these sections are frequently abundant in selections that are keto-friendly.

3. Prioritize Fresh Produce: Stock up on leafy greens and low-carb vegetables in the produce department. These nutrient-rich choices will give you fiber, vitamins, and minerals while limiting

the amount of carbohydrates you consume. To increase your intake of nutrients, aim for a diversity of hues.

4. Select High-Quality Proteins: Choose sources of protein that are of a high caliber, such as lean meats, poultry, fish, and shellfish. Whenever feasible, choose products that have been reared on grass or pastures. Avoid processed meats that could have additives or sugars hiding in them.

5. Choose Healthy Fats: Stock up on healthy fats such as nuts, seeds, avocados, olives, coconut oil, and olive oil. These will provide your body with the nourishment it needs and keep you full. Choose extra virgin or cold-pressed oils by reading labels.

6. Carefully read product labels to spot hidden sugars, components rich in carbohydrates, or unwholesome additions. Choose goods with little processing and elements that support your ketogenic objectives.

7. Limit processed foods because they frequently come with extra sugar, bad fats, and lots of carbohydrates. Limit your consumption of packaged foods, processed snacks, sugary drinks, and premade sauces. Focus on eating complete, unadulterated foods instead.

8. Be Wary of "Low-Carb" Products: Despite the abundance of low-carbohydrate foods on the market, some of them may not always adhere to the guidelines of a healthy ketogenic diet. Some high-processed or artificial sweetener-containing low-carb choices can have an impact on your insulin response and general health. When possible, choose entire foods.

9. The essentials for a keto pantry should be stored in your pantry, including coconut flour, almond flour, unsweetened nut butter, sugar replacements, and spices. When making keto-friendly meals and snacks, these will be useful.

10. Taking use of internet shopping options that let you filter and look for certain keto-friendly items is a good idea. By doing this, you may save time, avoid making impulsive purchases, and make sure you have everything you need to prepare your meals.

11. Plan for Meal Prep and Storage: Invest in high-quality food storage containers to keep your meals fresh and accessible if you intend to meal prep or batch cook. This will make going keto easier and make it easier for you to stay organized all week.

12. Don't Shop When Hungry: Shopping while hungry can result in impulsive buying of fatty, high-carb items. To avoid temptation, eat a filling keto-friendly snack before going to the grocery shop.

You can confidently shop at the grocery store and choose the best foods for your ketogenic diet by using these tactics and staying focused on your keto goals. Keep in mind that your success with the keto diet depends on the decisions you make at the grocery store.

Chapter 34: Tips for Batch Cooking and Meal Preparation

B atch cooking and meal planning are essential tactics for successfully following a ketogenic diet. You can save time, make sure you always have wholesome options on hand, and remain on track with your keto objectives by setting aside a few hours each week to plan and cook meals in advance. We will give you useful advice and pointers in this chapter to make meal planning and batch cooking effective and fun.

1. Plan Your Meals: Begin by making a weekly meal plan. Choose the recipes you wish to make and estimate the necessary serving sizes. Take into account your schedule and choose meals that can be quickly reheated or put together when you're pressed for time.

2. Recipes that are formulated specifically for the ketogenic diet should be chosen. There are several internet sources, cookbooks, and blogs that are keto-friendly that provide a variety of recipes to fit your interests. A good balance of protein, healthy fats, and low-carb vegetables should be present in the dishes.

3. Make a Shopping List: After choosing your recipes, make

a thorough shopping list. Make a list of the ingredients you currently have and the ones you need to buy. You can keep organized and cut down on last-minute food shop runs by doing this.

4. Set Aside Time: Each week, set aside a specified day or time for batch cooking and meal preparation. This could happen during the weekend or on a day when you have some free time. Schedule this time on your calendar as a priority to maintain consistency.

5. The first step in preparing the ingredients is to wash, chop, and portion your vegetables. When it comes to putting together your meals, this will save time. To speed up the cooking process, you can pre-cook some components like chicken, ground beef, or hard-boiled eggs.

6. Batch cooking is the process of making bigger amounts of food that may be divided into servings and kept for later use. Cook proteins in larger batches, such as chicken, beef, or fish. Additionally, you might roast a variety of low-carb vegetables or make a sizable pot of soup or stew that fits the keto diet.

7. Use reusable containers or meal prep containers to portion out your meals for portion control. You may maintain proper serving amounts and avoid overeating by doing this. Put the dish's name and the day it was made on the labels of the containers.

8. Storage and freezing: Keeping your prepared meals fresh and of high quality requires proper storage. You should freeze the remaining meals and put the ones you won't eat for a few days

in the refrigerator. To avoid freezer burn, use resealable bags or freezer-safe containers.

9. Think carefully about the best ways to reheat your prepared meals. While certain foods can be reheated in the microwave, others might need to be cooked on the stovetop or in the oven. To maintain flavor and texture, follow the suggested reheating directions for each meal.

10. Flexibility and diversity: To prevent boredom in your food planning, embrace variety. Every week, prepare a different meal to keep your taste buds happy. Additionally, make room in your meal plan for flexibility to account for shifting preferences or the discovery of new recipes.

11. Don't forget to prepare keto-friendly snacks when you're preparing your munchies. Into snack-sized containers, portion out nuts, seeds, cheese, or vegetables with dip. Having these on hand can make it easier for you to resist reaching for carb-heavy snacks when you get hungry.

12. Maintain Organization: Organize the ingredients and prepare meals in the refrigerator and freezer. Put them in a position that makes them accessible and guards against spoiling. Maintaining cleanliness and ensuring freshness requires routine cleaning of your storage containers.

Chapter 35: Recipes for Keto Newbies

I t can be intimidating to start a ketogenic diet, but with the correct recipes, you can do it confidently and with tasty food. We'll provide you with a variety of simple-to-make, tasty, and filling keto meals in this chapter that are suitable for beginners. These dishes will guide you through the beginning of your ketogenic diet and lay a solid basis for your future culinary explorations.

1. Eggs with avocado and bacon inside:
- Substances:
- 6 eggs, hard-boiled
1 mature avocado
- 3 crumbled slices of cooked bacon
- To taste, salt and pepper
- Requirements:
1. Remove the yolks from the hard-boiled eggs by cutting them in half lengthwise.

2. Mash the avocado in a bowl and stir in the crumbled bacon.

3. Add salt and pepper to taste.

4. Fill the egg white halves with the avocado and bacon mixture.

5. As a tasty and filling keto-friendly appetizer or snack, serve

cold.

2. Lemon-Garlic Chicken on the Grill:
   - Substances:
   - 4 skinless, boneless breasts of chicken
   - One lemon's juice
   - 2 minced garlic cloves
   Olive oil, 2 tablespoons
   - To taste, salt and pepper
   - Requirements:
   1. Set the grill's temperature to medium-high.
   2. Combine the lemon juice, garlic powder, olive oil, salt, and pepper in a small bowl.
   3. To ensure that the chicken breasts are thoroughly covered, brush the marinade over them.
   4. Cook the chicken on the preheated grill for 6 to 8 minutes on each side, or until the internal temperature reaches 165 degrees Fahrenheit (74 degrees Celsius).
   5. Before serving, take the chicken off the grill and allow it to rest for a while.
   6. For a whole keto-friendly supper, serve with a side of steamed veggies or a crisp salad.

3. Fried rice with cauliflower:
   - Substances:
   - 1 medium head of riced cauliflower
   -2 tbsp. sesame oil
   - 2 minced garlic cloves
   - 1 cup of mixed veggies, such as bell peppers, carrots, and peas
   - 2 tablespoons tamari (gluten-free alternative) or soy sauce

155

- 2 beaten eggs
- To taste, salt and pepper
- Requirements:

1. Sesame oil should be heated over medium heat in a sizable skillet or wok.

2. Sauté the minced garlic until fragrant after adding it.

3. Cook the mixed vegetables for a short while, until they start to soften.

4. Pour the beaten eggs onto the other side of the skillet, pushing the vegetables to one side.

5. The eggs should be well scrambled before being combined with the veggies.

6. When the cauliflower is heated through, add the riced cauliflower to the skillet and stir-fry for a few minutes.

7. Add salt and pepper to the cauliflower fried rice before drizzling soy sauce or tamari over it.

8. After thoroughly combining, simmer for one more minute.

9. Use as a tasty low-carb substitute for standard fried rice.

4. Salmon baked in a lemon butter sauce:
- Substances:
- 4 filets of salmon
- 4 teaspoons of melted butter
- One lemon's juice
- 2 minced garlic cloves
- To taste, salt and pepper
- Requirements:

1. Set the oven's temperature to 375°F (190°C).

2. Melted butter, lemon juice, minced garlic, salt, and pepper should all be combined in a small bowl.

3. Salmon filets should be put on a baking pan covered with

parchment paper.

4. Make sure to cover each piece of salmon with the lemon butter sauce.

5. Bake the salmon for 12 to 15 minutes, or until it is cooked through and flakes easily.

6. For a filling and healthy keto-friendly lunch, serve the baked salmon with steamed asparagus or a green salad.

5. Chicken Breast Stuffed with Spinach and Feta:
   - Substances:
   - 4 skinless, boneless breasts of chicken
   - 2 cups chopped fresh spinach
   - 1/2 cup feta cheese, crumbled
   - 2 minced garlic cloves
   Olive oil, 2 tablespoons
   - To taste, salt and pepper
   - Requirements:
   1. Set the oven's temperature to 400°F (200°C).
   2. Olive oil should be heated in a skillet over medium heat.
   3. Sauté the minced garlic until fragrant after adding it.
   4. To the skillet, add the spinach, and cook until wilted.
   5. Remove spinach from the heat and let it cool slightly.
   6. Add the feta cheese crumbles and season with salt and pepper.
   7. Each chicken breast has a pocket that can be cut out and filled with the feta and spinach mixture.
   8. If necessary, close the gaps with toothpicks.
   9. Bake the stuffed chicken breasts for 20 to 25 minutes, or until the chicken is well done.
   10. Serve alongside a fresh salad or roasted vegetables for a tasty and protein-heavy keto dinner.

6. Noodles of zucchini in a creamy garlic-parmesan sauce:
- Substances:
- 2 medium zucchinis made into noodles by spiralizing them
butter, 2 tablespoons
- 2 minced garlic cloves
half a cup of heavy cream
- One-fourth cup of grated Parmesan cheese
- To taste, salt and pepper
- Requirements:
1. Melt the butter in a large skillet over medium heat.
2. Sauté the minced garlic until fragrant after adding it.
3. Cook the zucchini noodles in the skillet for two to three minutes, or until they start to soften.
4. Add the grated Parmesan cheese and heavy cream.
5. After thoroughly combining it, simmer the sauce for a few minutes to thicken it.
6. To taste, add salt and pepper to the food.
7. As a tasty and low-carb alternative to pasta, remove from heat and serve the zucchini noodles with the creamy garlic Parmesan sauce.

7. Avocado and Chocolate Smoothie:
- Substances:
1 mature avocado
- 1 cup almond milk that is unsweetened
- 2 tablespoons chocolate powder, unsweetened
- 1 teaspoon of almond butter
- Optional 1 tablespoon sweetener, such as erythritol or stevia
- If desired, ice cubes
- Requirements:
1. Blend the ripe avocado with the almond milk, chocolate,

almond butter, and sweetener, if using, in a blender.

2. Blend till creamy and smooth.

3. To get the consistency you want, add ice cubes and combine once more.

4. Pour into a glass, and indulge in a decadent and filling chocolate avocado smoothie as a low-carb dessert or snack.

These dishes serve as a jumping-off point for your culinary study of the keto diet. To fit your taste preferences, feel free to experiment with various tastes, spices, and ingredients. To make sure they support your keto goals, don't forget to track your macros and portion amounts. With the help of these delectable and easy-to-follow keto recipes, enjoy your transition to a healthier way of life.

Chapter 36: Advanced Keto Recipes for Variety

It's time to investigate sophisticated dishes that will increase your cooking abilities as you grow more accustomed to the ketogenic diet. These recipes use a wider variety of ingredients, flavors, and cooking methods, giving you more alternatives for keto meals and a wider selection of foods to choose from. This chapter will expose you to several sophisticated ketogenic dishes that will satiate your palate and provide you access to tasty and varied keto cuisine.

1. Baked salmon with lemon butter sauce and dill:
    - Substances:
    - 4 filets of salmon
    - 4 teaspoons of melted butter
    - One lemon's juice
    - 2 teaspoons finely chopped fresh dill
    - To taste, salt and pepper
    - Requirements:
    1. Set the oven's temperature to 375°F (190°C).
    2. Salmon filets should be put on a baking pan covered with parchment paper.
    3. Melted butter, lemon juice, minced dill, salt, and pepper

should all be combined in a small basin.

4. Make sure to cover each piece of salmon with the dill and lemon butter sauce.

5. Bake the salmon for 12 to 15 minutes, or until it is cooked through and flakes easily.

6. For a chic and savory keto lunch, serve the baked salmon with a side of roasted asparagus or cauliflower rice.

2. Pizza with cauliflower crust:
  - Substances:
  - To make the crust
  - 1 medium head of riced cauliflower
  - 1/2 cup of finely grated Parmesan cheese
  - Shredded half a cup of mozzarella cheese
  1 tsp. dried oregano
  - Half a teaspoon of garlic powder
  - 2 beaten eggs
  - To taste, salt and pepper
  - For the garnishes
  - Low-carb tomato sauce or marinara sauce
  - Shredded mozzarella cheese
  - A variety of veggies, including bell peppers, onions, and mushrooms
  - Chopped cooked bacon
  - Fresh leaves of basil

- Requirements:
  1. Set the oven's temperature to 425°F (220°C).
  2. In a bowl that can go in the microwave, place the riced cauliflower and microwave for 5 minutes.
  3. The cauliflower should be moved to a clean kitchen towel

and squeezed to remove as much liquid as you can after cooling.

4. Cauliflower, grated Parmesan, shredded mozzarella, dried oregano, garlic powder, beaten eggs, salt, and pepper should all be combined in a mixing bowl.

5. Mix thoroughly until dough-like consistency develops.

6. Place the cauliflower dough in the shape of a pizza crust on a baking pan covered with parchment paper.

7. The crust should be baked in the preheated oven for 12 to 15 minutes, or until golden brown.

8. Spread a thin layer of tomato sauce on the crust after taking it out of the oven.

9. Add cooked bacon, chopped vegetables, and mozzarella cheese on top.

10. Once more, bake the pizza in the oven for 10 to 12 more minutes, or until the cheese is melted and bubbling.

11. Before serving, garnish with fresh basil leaves. Enjoy a tasty keto-friendly pizza substitute.

3. Stir-fry with beef and broccoli:
   - Substances:
   - 1 pound of thinly sliced beef sirloin or flank steak
   - 3 tablespoons of soy sauce or tamari
   Olive oil, 2 tablespoons
   - 3 minced garlic cloves
   - 2 teaspoons grated fresh ginger
   - 1 broccoli head, separated into florets
   - 1/4 cup water or beef broth
   -2 tbsp. sesame oil
   - To taste, salt and pepper

- Requirements:

1. Tamari or soy sauce should be used to marinate the thinly sliced beef for 15 to 20 minutes in a bowl.

2. In a big skillet or wok, heat the olive oil over high heat.

3. Stir-fry the grated ginger and minced garlic in the skillet for one minute.

4. When the beef is added to the skillet, brown it on all sides.

5. From the skillet, take out the beef, and set it aside.

6. Broccoli florets and beef broth or water should be added to the same skillet.

7. The broccoli should be tender-crisp after 3–4 minutes of cooking under cover.

8. Add the sesame oil and put the steak back in the skillet.

9. To taste, add salt and pepper to the food.

10. To give the flavors a chance to mingle, stir-fry for a further two to three minutes.

11. As a tasty and filling keto supper option, serve the beef and broccoli stir-fry.

4. Noodles with Spicy Shrimp and Zucchini:
   - Substances:
   - One pound of peeled and deveined shrimp
   Olive oil, 2 tablespoons
   - 3 minced garlic cloves
   - 1 teaspoon chili flakes (modify to your level of heat)
   - 3 medium zucchinis made into noodles by spiralizing them
   - One-fourth cup of chicken broth
   - To taste, salt and pepper

- Requirements:
   1. In a large skillet over medium-high heat, warm the olive oil.

2. To the skillet, add the minced garlic and chili flakes, and cook for one minute.

3. Add the shrimp to the skillet and cook for 3–4 minutes on each side, or until pink and opaque.

4. The shrimp should be taken out of the skillet and put aside.

5. Add the chicken stock and zucchini noodles to the same skillet.

6. The noodles should be sautéed for two to three minutes, or until they start to soften.

7. Zucchini noodles are tossed with the shrimp once they have been added back to the skillet.

8. To taste, add salt and pepper to the food.

9. To fully heat everything, continue cooking for one more minute.

10. As a tasty and low-carb substitute for typical pasta dishes, serve spicy shrimp and zucchini noodles.

5. Suitable Beef Stroganoff for Ketosis:
   - Substances:
   - 1 pound of thinly sliced beef sirloin
   butter, 2 tablespoons
   - 1 thinly sliced tiny onion
   - 8 ounces of sliced mushrooms
   - 2 minced garlic cloves
   - One cup of beef broth
   - Half a cup of sour cream
   2-tablespoons of Dijon mustard
   - To taste, salt and pepper

- Requirements:
   1. In a large skillet over medium heat, melt the butter.

2. The beef strips should be added to the skillet and cooked for 3–4 minutes on each side, or until browned.

3. From the skillet, take out the beef, and set it aside.

4. Add the diced onion and mushrooms to the same skillet.

5. About 5 to 6 minutes of sautéing will soften the vegetables and cause the mushrooms to lose their liquid.

6. To the skillet, add the minced garlic, and cook for one more minute.

7. Add the beef broth, then boil the mixture.

8. Sour cream and Dijon mustard should be thoroughly mixed in.

9. For two to three minutes, add the steak back to the skillet and heat everything through.

10. To taste, add salt and pepper to the food.

11. Give the keto-friendly beef stroganoff a plate of steamed vegetables or serve it over cauliflower rice.

6. Chicken Breast Stuffed with Bacon:
   - Substances:
   - 4 skinless, boneless breasts of chicken
   - 4 ounces softened cream cheese
   - One-fourth cup of grated Parmesan cheese
   - 2 teaspoons of freshly chopped herbs, such as chives, basil, or parsley
   - 8 bacon slices
   - To taste, salt and pepper

- Requirements:
   1. Set the oven's temperature to 375°F (190°C).
   2. Melted cream cheese, grated Parmesan cheese, chopped fresh herbs, salt, and pepper should all be combined in a bowl.

165

3. Each chicken breast is given a pocket that is to be filled with the cheese and cream mixture.

4. Two slices of bacon are wrapped around each packed chicken breast, and if necessary, they are fastened with toothpicks.

5. On a baking sheet covered with parchment paper, put the chicken breasts that have been wrapped in bacon.

6. Bake for 25 to 30 minutes, or until the chicken is cooked through and the bacon is crisp, in the preheated oven.

7. Before serving, take the toothpicks out.

8. For a tasty and filling keto supper, serve the bacon-wrapped stuffed chicken breast with roasted vegetables on the side or a crisp salad.

These sophisticated keto recipes will improve your culinary abilities and provide you access to a wide variety of tastes and textures. They demonstrate the adaptability of the ketogenic diet and how you might take pleasure in scrumptious foods while leading a low-carb lifestyle. Put on your chef's hat, investigate these recipes, and enjoy the satisfaction of producing dishes of restaurant quality right in your home kitchen.

Your taste buds will be wowed by these sophisticated keto recipes, which will liven up your keto meal plan. They show that you may follow a ketogenic diet and yet appreciate a variety of tastes and sensations. So get your hands dirty, try these recipes, and enjoy the flavor of sophisticated keto cooking.

Chapter 37: Challenges Overcome: Overcoming Keto Flu and Plateaus

S tarting a ketogenic diet can have a lot of great effects on your body and your health, but like any lifestyle change, it can also present some difficulties. This chapter will discuss the keto flu and plateaus, two major obstacles that people following the ketogenic diet may experience. To help you remain on track and accomplish your goals, we'll examine the origins, signs, and solutions to these problems.

1. **Recognizing the Keto Flu**

The "keto flu" is a transitory series of symptoms that some people may experience while starting a ketogenic diet as their bodies get used to burning fat as their main fuel source rather than carbohydrates. Fatigue, headaches, irritability, nausea, dizziness, and brain fog are a few possible symptoms.

Electrolyte imbalances and dehydration brought on by the body's abrupt switch in fuel sources are typical causes of the keto flu. Considering the following tactics will help you recover from the keto flu:

a. Stay Hydrated: Drink more water to support your body's

electrolyte balance and appropriate hydration. Drink electrolyte-rich liquids, such as electrolyte-enhanced water or sugar-free sports drinks, or add a pinch of sea salt to your water.

b. Increase Your Intake of Electrolytes: Eat More Electrolyte-Rich Foods Like Avocados, Leafy Greens, Nuts, and Seeds. Magnesium, potassium, and salt supplements are also available as needed; however, before beginning any new supplements, seek the advice of a healthcare provider.

c. Reduce Your Carbohydrate Intake Gradually: Instead of suddenly eliminating all carbohydrates, cut back on them gradually over a few days or weeks. This can lessen how bad the symptoms get as your body gets used to being in a ketogenic condition.

d. Adequate Sleep and relaxation: During the first period of transition, give your body enough time to relax and heal. Give excellent sleep a high priority to enhance your general well-being and help you through the adjustment period.

2. **Moving Beyond Stalls:**
Even though the ketogenic diet can result in significant weight loss and better metabolic health, plateaus are frequently encountered. These halts or slowdowns in weight reduction happen as your body acclimates to the new eating habits and reaches this point. A strategic approach is necessary to get over plateaus:

a. Make sure you are still in a calorie deficit and that your macronutrient ratios are in line with your objectives. Reevaluate your macros. If required, recalculate your daily caloric intake and change your ratios of fat, protein, and carbohydrates.

b. Track Your Intake: Track your food intake in great detail and keep an eye on your portion proportions. Progress can be hampered by unintentionally consuming extra calories or carbohydrates that are not readily apparent.

c. Consider Intermittent Fasting: By allowing your body more time to use stored fat as energy, intermittent fasting can help you get beyond plateaus. Try out various fasting programs to determine which one suits you the best.

d. Modify Your Exercise Program: Review Your Program. Your metabolism can be revitalized and supported by adding new workouts, upping the intensity, or including weight training.

e. Maintain Your Consistency and Patience: Any weight reduction journey will inevitably experience plateaus. Maintain your dedication to the ketogenic diet, be patient, and have faith in the process. Keep in mind that development is not always linear and that your body might simply require some time to adjust before you can resume losing weight.

examining other ways to address these issues:

3. Taking Care of the Keto Flu
   a. Put electrolyte balance first because it's a common cause of the keto flu. Increase your consumption of foods high in electrolytes such as avocados, leafy greens, nuts, and seeds. Consider taking supplements that contain magnesium, potas-

sium, and sodium as well. However, before beginning any new supplements, seek the advice of a healthcare provider.

b. Keep Hydrated: Staying properly hydrated is essential for both preventing and treating the keto flu's symptoms. Drink enough water throughout the day, and think about adding a pinch of sea salt or sipping beverages with added electrolytes.

c. Adequate Fat and Caloric Intake: During the transition, make sure you are getting enough healthy fats to meet your body's energy needs. to avoid extreme calorie restriction, which might worsen the symptoms, adjust your caloric intake as needed.

d. Give Your Body Time: Recognize that the keto flu is typically transient and that it will go away as your body becomes used to being in a ketogenic state. Give your body the time it requires to adjust, and practice patience with yourself.

4. Moving Beyond Stalls:

a. Review Your Macros: **Reexamine your calor**ie intake and macronutrient ratios. If your body has acclimated to your current eating strategy, changing your macronutrient ratios may help you lose weight again. To determine which combination of fats, proteins, and carbohydrates is optimal for your body, experiment with different ratios.

b. Include Intermittent Fasting: By causing a calorie deficit and encouraging fat burning, intermittent fasting can aid in overcoming plateaus. Find a timetable that works for your lifestyle by researching several fasting protocols, such as the 16/8 approach or alternate-day fasting.

c. Focus on entire Foods: Make sure that the majority of the ingredients in your meals are entire, nutrient-dense foods. Focus on including a variety of veggies, lean meats, healthy fats, and low-carb fruits in your meals instead of processed foods.

d. Change Up Your Training Routine: Add a variety of exercises to your training plan to keep things interesting. You can boost your metabolism and encourage weight loss by engaging in high-intensity interval training (HIIT), strength training, or trying out new exercise classes.

e. Control your stress levels because they can impede your efforts to lose weight. Incorporate stress-reduction strategies like yoga, deep breathing exercises, meditation, or indulging in your favorite pastimes.

f. Join local or online support groups to meet people who are also following the ketogenic diet. Sharing stories, advice, and tactics can inspire and encourage people to move past obstacles.

Remember, you must have patience, tenacity, and the willingness to change your strategy to get over the keto flu and break past plateaus. You'll be better able to overcome these obstacles and keep moving forward on your path to greater health and well-being if you put these techniques into practice and maintain your ketogenic lifestyle.

Keep your resolve, your attention, and your enthusiasm for overcoming challenges as they come. You can succeed on the ketogenic diet if you have the correct attitude and strategies in place.

171

Chapter 38: Exercise While Following a Ketogenic Diet

To maintain overall health and support the ketogenic way of life, exercise is essential. In this chapter, we will examine the advantages of working out while on a ketogenic diet, go through the pros and downsides of various forms of exercise, and offer helpful advice for getting the most out of your workouts.

On a ketogenic diet, exercise has several advantages.

When paired with a ketogenic diet, regular exercise has several benefits:

a. Increased Fat Burning: Physical activity can help your body burn fat that is stored as fuel more efficiently. Exercise and a low-carbohydrate diet work together to enhance fat adaption, which boosts the effectiveness of fat metabolism.

b. Exercise promotes the growth of lean muscle mass while also lowering body fat, which results in improvements in body composition. This may lead to a body that is more defined and toned.

c. Enhanced Energy and Endurance: As your body adjusts to using fat as a fuel source, you can notice heightened energy and enhanced endurance while working out. Long-lasting workout sessions can be sustained by the constant flow of energy provided by ketones.

d. Improved Metabolic Health: A ketogenic diet and exercise can enhance insulin sensitivity, control blood sugar levels, and promote metabolic health as a whole. Regular exercise has been associated with a lower chance of developing chronic conditions like diabetes, cardiovascular disease, and obesity.

e. Mental Health: Exercise has been shown to improve mood, lower stress levels, and sharpen the mind. Exercise's endorphin release and the neuroprotective properties of the ketogenic diet can work together to improve mental health.

2. Exercise and Ketogenic Diet Considerations:
   Keep the following things in mind when combining exercise into your ketogenic diet:

a. Hydration: It's important to be properly hydrated, especially when on a low-carbohydrate diet. you stay hydrated, make sure you drink enough water before, during, and after exercise.

b. Electrolyte Balance: When exercising and eating a ketogenic diet, electrolyte imbalances can happen, especially during strenuous workouts. Consume foods high in electrolytes or, if necessary, think about taking supplements of sodium, potassium, and magnesium.

173

c. Meal Timing: Take into account the timing of your meals and your workouts. While some people prefer to exercise while fasting, others might benefit from having a modest pre-workout snack. Try out various strategies to see which suits your body the best.

d. Muscle repair and protein intake: Getting enough protein is essential for these processes. Make sure you're getting adequate sources of high-quality protein to help your muscles grow and heal.

e. Gradual Adaptation: Give your body time to get used to both exercise and the ketogenic diet if you're new to them. As your level of fitness increases, progressively up the intensity and duration of your workouts from moderate to vigorous.

3. Advice for Working Out While Following a Ketogenic Diet:
To maximize the effectiveness and outcomes of your workouts, take into account the following helpful advice:

a. Fuel with Healthy Fats: Make healthy fats, such as those found in avocados, nuts, seeds, and olive oil, your main source of energy. These fats support the formation of ketone during exercise and offer steady energy.

b. Consume Foods High in Protein: Consume enough protein to aid in the maintenance and repair of your muscles. Include sources of protein in your meals such as lean meats, poultry, fish, eggs, and plant-based protein alternatives.

c. Focus on low-impact cardiovascular workouts, such as

walking, cycling, swimming, or utilizing an elliptical machine. c. Without placing an undue amount of strain on your joints, these activities can efficiently burn calories.

d. Incorporate Strength Training: To develop and maintain lean muscle mass, incorporate resistance training activities into your workout program. Strength training is beneficial promotes general strength, increases metabolism, and enhances body composition.

e. Listen to Your Body: Pay attention to your body's signals and modify the intensity and length of your workouts as necessary. To avoid overtraining and injuries, give yourself enough time to relax and recover between workouts.

f. Monitor Your Progress: Keep a log of your workouts, noting the exercises done, their length, and their difficulty. This will enable you to monitor your advancement over time and make any adjustments.

g. Seek Professional Advice: If you're new to training or have special fitness objectives, think about hiring a licensed personal trainer or other fitness expert. They may make customized training plans, offer targeted advice, and guarantee correct form and technique.

When it comes to exercising while following a ketogenic diet, consistency is essential. Find long-lasting activities that you can sustain. You'll optimize the advantages and reach your health and fitness goals by combining regular exercise with a well-formulated ketogenic diet.

Chapter 39: Supplements that Aid Your Keto Journey are Covered

Even while a well-designed ketogenic diet can give you all the nutrients you need, several supplements can improve your overall health and make the most of your keto adventure. In this chapter, we'll look at some of the supplements that are frequently suggested for those following the ketogenic diet, their advantages, and how they might support your dietary goals.

1. Electrolyte supplements: It's important to maintain electrolyte balance, particularly while switching to a ketogenic diet. You may have an increased excretion of electrolytes like salt, potassium, and magnesium since ketosis has a diuretic impact. These vital elements can be replenished and imbalances prevented with the aid of electrolyte supplements. A balanced amount of sodium, potassium, and magnesium should be present in the electrolyte powders or capsules you choose.

2. Omega-3 Fatty Acids: Essential fats, notably EPA (eicosapentaenoic acid) and DHA (docosahexaenoic acid), play a critical role in maintaining the health of the heart, the brain, and the body by lowering inflammation. Although fatty fish like

salmon and mackerel are great sources of omega-3s, taking high-quality fish oil or algae-based omega-3 supplements can be helpful, particularly if you don't eat fish often.

3. MCT Oil: People following a ketogenic diet can use medium-chain triglycerides (MCTs), a form of fat, as an easy source of energy. MCTs are a type of fat that is readily converted into ketones. To improve your intake of these easily accessible ketone precursors, you can add MCT oil, which is made from coconut or palm kernel oil to your meals or beverages. MCT oil can support fat burning, increase energy levels, and improve mental clarity.

4. Exogenous Ketones: To raise blood ketone levels, one can take exogenous ketones as a supplement. They are not necessary for a successful ketogenic diet, however, they may come in handy occasionally. Exogenous ketones are frequently utilized to improve mental clarity, provide workout participants with an energy boost, or smooth the transition into ketosis. They can be taken as a drink or supplement and come in the form of ketone salts or ketone esters.

5. Fiber supplements: Getting enough fiber is important for a healthy digestive system and regular bowel motions. Even while many plant-based foods included in a ketogenic diet are naturally high in fiber, some people can benefit from taking additional fiber supplements. Look for fiber supplements made from materials like glucomannan, psyllium husk, or acacia fiber. These vitamins can encourage satiety, improve gut health, and control bowel motions.

6. Multivitamin and Mineral Supplements: Even though a well-designed ketogenic diet can offer a variety of nutrients, some people may still gain from taking a high-quality multivitamin and mineral supplement. This can ensure that you get the necessary amounts of vitamins and minerals each day, especially if you have tight dietary requirements or few food options. Look for a complete supplement made for people following a ketogenic or low-carb diet.

7. Adaptogenic Herbs and Supplements: Adaptogens are herbal and dietary products that can aid in the body's ability to adjust to stress and foster general well-being. While adaptogens like ashwagandha, Rhodiola rosea, or holy basil are not specifically for a ketogenic diet, they can support your body's stress response, help with hormonal balance, and foster a sense of calm and relaxation.

8. Probiotics: A balanced gut microbiome is essential for digestion and overall health. A broad and healthy gut microbiota can be supported with probiotics, which are helpful microorganisms. While yogurt, kimchi, and other fermented foods are natural sources of probiotics, taking a high-quality probiotic supplement might be helpful, particularly if you have certain digestive problems or have recently used antibiotics.

9. Vitamin D: Vitamin D is a necessary nutrient that is vital for the immune system and overall health as well as bone health. While vitamin D can be produced by the body when exposed to sunlight, many people may not have appropriate amounts, particularly in the winter or for those who get a little sun. Vitamin D3 supplements can assist maintain ideal levels and

support several physiological processes.

10. Magnesium: A mineral necessary for energy synthesis, muscle contraction, and many enzymatic processes in the body, magnesium is a vital mineral. It contributes to keeping blood pressure levels at a healthy range. Due to the increased excretion of magnesium through urine, some people following a ketogenic diet may have a deficit in this mineral. You can help achieve your daily magnesium requirements by taking supplements of magnesium citrate, magnesium glycinate, or magnesium oxide.

11. Collagen: The most prevalent protein in the body, collagen gives tissues including the skin, joints, and bones structural stability. Collagen peptides and hydrolyzed collagen supplements help improve joint health, skin elasticity, and potential hair and nail growth. For an additional protein boost, collagen is readily blended into drinks or added to dishes.

12. Green tea extract: Green tea extract is rich in catechins, potent antioxidants that have been linked to several health advantages. They might improve metabolism, promote weight loss, and have neuroprotective properties. To take advantage of the possible advantages, green tea extract can be eaten as a supplement or as a beverage.

13. Prebiotic Fiber: Prebiotic fiber provides food for the good bacteria in your gut, helping to maintain a balanced microbiome there. Prebiotic fiber supplements, like inulin or chicory root fiber, can support digestive health, promote regular bowel movements, and improve nutrient absorption. To prevent gastric pain, it's crucial to start with a modest dosage and raise

it gradually.

14. Sleeping pills: Getting enough sleep is crucial for one's general health and well-being. Certain supplements, such as melatonin or magnesium, can support restful sleep promotion and cycle regulation. Prioritizing sound sleep practices and seeking medical advice for any underlying sleep problems are nevertheless crucial.

15. Carnitine: A substance that transports fatty acids into the mitochondria, where they are turned into energy, is known as carnitine. Acetyl-L-carnitine, often known as L-carnitine, is a supplement that can promote energy generation, improve athletic performance, and help with fat burning. As it might help maximize the use of fat as fuel, it may be especially advantageous for people on the ketogenic diet.

16. Chromium: This mineral is important for the metabolism of glucose and insulin. It might lessen cravings for carbohydrates and manage blood sugar levels. Chromium picolinate or chromium polynicotinate supplements can help people manage their blood sugar levels in a healthy way, especially those who have insulin resistance or are trying to lose weight.

17. Coenzyme Q10 (CoQ10): Coenzyme Q10 is an antioxidant and naturally occurring substance that is used in the creation of cellular energy. It can improve exercise performance, defend against oxidative stress, and support heart health. Because they are eating fewer of some items, people on a ketogenic diet may have low levels of CoQ10. Taking CoQ10 supplements can promote overall vigor and help keep levels at their ideal levels.

18. Berberine: A natural substance that can be found in a variety of plants and may have health benefits, berberine has been used in traditional medicine. It might support weight management, control blood sugar levels, and enhance cardiovascular health. To improve metabolic health and enhance the effects of a ketogenic diet, berberine can be used as a supplement.

19. Ashwagandha: For thousands of years, Ayurvedic medicine has used the adaptogenic herb ashwagandha. It might aid in lowering tension, encouraging relaxation, and supporting general well-being. Ashwagandha supplements, which are frequently standardized for withanolide content, can be helpful for people who are suffering from symptoms associated with stress or who want to strengthen their mental and emotional resilience while on the ketogenic diet.

20. Digestive Enzymes: For people with digestive problems or those starting a ketogenic diet, digestive enzymes can help with healthy digestion and nutrition absorption. A broad-spectrum digestive enzyme supplement that contains amylase, protease, and lipase can aid in the breakdown of macronutrients and enhance digestive health.

It's crucial to remember that while supplements might be beneficial, a nutrient-dense diet should always come first. Focus on whole, natural foods as the cornerstone of your ketogenic diet, and use supplements to round out your nutritional efforts and take care of particular needs. Before beginning any new supplements, always check with a medical expert or certified nutritionist to make sure they are suitable for your unique health and circumstances.

You may optimize your nutritional intake, support particular elements of your health, and improve the overall efficacy of your ketogenic lifestyle by including these supplements in your ketogenic journey. For the best outcomes, keep in mind to prefer reliable brands and adhere to suggested dosages.

Chapter 40: Eating Out and Traveling on Keto: Staying Social

How to deal with social circumstances, such as dining out or traveling, while adhering to your nutritional goals is one of the major worries when on a ketogenic diet. This chapter will cover methods and advice for keeping up a ketogenic diet while taking part in social activities and traveling to new locations.

1. Eating Out on Keto: Going out to eat doesn't have to be difficult when following a ketogenic diet. You can make keto-friendly decisions and still eat tasty food with a little forethought and understanding. Observe the following advice:

A. Research the Menu: Spend some time online researching the menu before visiting a restaurant. to accommodate your dietary requirements, look for recipes that are naturally low in carbohydrates. Choose meats that have been roasted or grilled, seafood, salads that are high in protein and healthy fats, and non-starchy vegetables. Steer clear of foods that are fried, breaded, or have high-carb sauces and dressings.

b. Tailor Your Order: Don't be hesitant to request changes

to meet your keto specifications. Ask for alternatives such as extra vegetables in place of carbohydrates like rice or potatoes, dressing on the side, or sauces without added sugars. The majority of eateries are accommodating and will be pleased to fulfill your wishes.

c. Be Aware of Hidden Carbs: Watch out for condiments, sauces, and marinades that may be hiding carbohydrates. These might interfere with your ketogenic aims if they have extra sugars or starches. Request that these be left off the menu or served on the side.

d. Choose Keto-Friendly Drinks: Select sugar-free beverages like sparkling water, unsweetened tea, or coffee. Avoid fruit juices, alcoholic drinks with lots of carbs, and sugary soft drinks. If you do decide to drink, go for tequila, vodka, or rum diluted with soda water or other sugar-free mixers.

2. Traveling while on a ketogenic diet may require a little more preparation, but it is doable to adhere to your nutritional objectives. Here are some tips to keep up your ketogenic diet while you're away from home:

a. Bring portable keto-friendly snacks: Get ready in advance by taking along portable keto-friendly snacks. Low-carb protein bars, nuts, seeds, beef jerky, cheese sticks, and other accessible options can keep you full and deter you from reaching for high-carb snacks.

b. Look up Local Restaurants: Do some research on nearby eateries or markets that have keto-friendly selections before you go. Seek out restaurants that provide grilled meats, salads, or vegetable-based meals. Finding nearby eateries that cater to the keto diet can be facilitated by using apps and websites like Yelp and TripAdvisor.

c. Choosing keto-friendly foods should be a priority when eating out or getting takeout while traveling. Healthy fats and non-starchy veggies should also be included. Choose meats, fish, salads, and vegetable sides that have been grilled or roasted. Keto-friendly options are available in many different cuisines, including grilled kebabs, stir-fries, and seafood dishes.

d. Prepare in Advance for Air Travel: If you're flying, you must prepare your in-flight meals and snacks in advance. Most airlines allow you to bring your meals or choose low-carb options. Prepare travel-friendly meals or snacks, such as hard-boiled eggs, bacon that has already been cooked, or sliced veggies with a dipping sauce.

e. Maintain Hydration: Traveling can occasionally cause dehydration, so be sure to drink plenty of water the entire way. Carry a reusable water bottle, and drink enough fluids, especially if you're going somewhere hot or doing physical activity.

f. Express Your Dietary Needs: Don't be afraid to let the restaurant staff or event planners know if you have special dietary requirements when you're out to eat or attending social gatherings. Mentioning your ketogenic diet and politely requesting modifications or recommendations for keto-friendly options. Many eateries and businesses are prepared to work with you to provide a delicious meal as they become more conscious of various dietary requirements.

g. Exercise Portion Control: When eating out, portions are frequently bigger than what you would normally eat. Eat mindfully and pay attention to your body's signals of hunger and fullness. If you want to store leftovers for later, think about sharing a dish with a buddy or ordering a takeaway container. You can maintain your desired calorie and macronutrient consumption by being cautious of portion sizes.

h. Keep Moving: It's crucial to keep moving while following a ketogenic diet. When you're traveling, take advantage of the chance to walk around and investigate your surroundings or partake in enjoyable physical activities. Look for nearby parks or gyms that provide exercise opportunities. Maintaining an active lifestyle can help you achieve your fitness objectives as well as enhance your general well-being.

i. Prepare for Emergencies: It's always a good idea to have a fallback plan in case there aren't enough or no keto-friendly options available. Take into account packing some portable, simple-to-store keto-friendly snacks or meal substitutes. This way, if you ever find yourself in a scenario where there aren't many options for suitable food, you'll have a backup plan.

J. accept Flexibility: While adhering to your ketogenic lifestyle is important, it's also crucial to accept flexibility and avoid being unduly anxious about each dietary choice. Take in the social aspects of eating out and traveling while concentrating on selecting the best options that are available to you. Keep in mind that one meal or one day off from your usual keto diet won't undo all your hard work. With your subsequent meal, go back on track and keep up your ketogenic diet.

By using these techniques, you can successfully handle social situations, enjoy eating out, and travel while maintaining your ketogenic diet. Keep in mind that keeping on track and making the most of these events without jeopardizing your nutritional objectives requires planning, communicating, and monitoring.

Take advantage of the chance to try new tastes, cuisines, and activities while adhering to your ketogenic ideals throughout your journey. You can strike a healthy balance between your devotion to a ketogenic lifestyle and your love of socializing with some effort and a positive outlook.

Chapter 41: Maintaining Long-Term Success

Having arrived at this stage in your ketogenic journey, congratulations! It's crucial to concentrate on tactics that will enable you to maintain your progress as you move forward on your path to long-term success and turn the ketogenic diet into a sustainable and pleasurable way of life. We will examine important elements for sustaining long-term success on a ketogenic diet in this chapter.

1. Consistency is Key: Following a ketogenic diet consistently is essential for long-term success. Aim to continuously adhere to the principles of a well-designed ketogenic diet, which include moderate consumption of protein, a high intake of healthy fats, and a low intake of carbohydrates. Recurrent slip-ups or dieting up and down can throw off your body's adaptation to ketosis and impede your success.

2. Regular Monitoring and Adjustments: Keep tabs on your progress by periodically gauging your energy levels, body composition, and general well-being. To make sure you're on track, monitor your macronutrient intake, ketone levels, and any other pertinent health indicators. Make any necessary adjustments

to maximize your outcomes based on your findings. This can entail altering your calorie consumption, experimenting with various meal options, or shifting your macronutrient ratios.

3. Mindful Eating: Develop a positive relationship with food by engaging in mindful eating, which will also enhance your whole dining experience. Pay attention to your body's signals of hunger and satiety, and consume food until you are contentedly full. Savor each bite, pay attention to the quality of your food choices, and be present when you eat. To enjoy your meals to the fullest, refrain from using screens or multitasking while you're eating.

4. Regular Physical Activity: To promote your general health and well-being, include regular physical activity in your daily routine. Exercise your cardiovascular system, your muscles, and your flexibility at the same time. Make enjoyable activities a regular part of your life by finding them. Along with helping with weight management, exercise also benefits bone density, cardiovascular health, and mental wellness.

5. Emotional Well-Being: Your emotional well-being is important to your long-term success, so pay attention to it. Find good coping mechanisms for stress, such as mindfulness training, relaxation techniques, or engaging in interests and pursuits that make you happy. Make sure you have a network of friends and family who accept and understand your food preferences.

6. Seek Professional Assistance: Take into account collaborating with a medical expert, licensed dietitian, or nutritionist who is knowledgeable about ketogenic diets. They may offer you

individualized advice, assist you in resolving problems, and make sure your nutrient requirements are being met. They can also help you with any particular health issues or objectives you may have.

7. Lifelong Learning: Maintain your curiosity and keep learning more about diet, health, and the science of the ketogenic diet. Follow the most recent findings by reading publications, watching documentaries, listening to podcasts, and attending conferences and seminars on low-carb and ketogenic diets. You will be equipped to make wise judgments and maintain your motivation as you progress thanks to this ongoing education.

8. Flexibility and Adaptability: Keep in mind that there is no one-size-fits-all approach to the ketogenic diet. Be willing to modify and alter your dietary strategy by your own needs, tastes, and objectives. Finding the ketogenic diet that is right for you, whether it be strict keto, cyclical keto, or focused keto, is crucial. Maintain your adaptability and willingness to adjust for the sake of your long-term sustainability and satisfaction.

9. Celebrate Successes Away From the Scale: Even if losing weight may be one of your goals, don't limit your attention to that number. Celebrate your successes that don't include the scale, such as increased energy, mental clarity, better sleep, better digestion, or better-fitting clothes. These accomplishments are equally significant markers of your general well-being and development.

10. Have Fun on the Road: Last but not least, have fun on the road. Accept the range of delectable things that you can eat

when following a ketogenic diet. Discover new recipes, try out various flavors and ingredients, and talk to others about your experiences. Concentrate on the benefits of a ketogenic diet for your health and the joy it provides to your life.

You may sustain long-term success on your ketogenic journey by adopting these techniques into your daily life. Maintain consistency, pay attention to your body, care for your emotional health, and never stop learning and evolving. Keep in mind that adopting a ketogenic diet and lifestyle is a long-term strategy for nourishing your body and improving your health. It is not a quick fix.

Printed in Great Britain
by Amazon